The

Illusion

of

Certainty

[Health Benefits and Risks]

The
Illusion
of
Certainty

[Health Benefits and Risks]

Erik Rifkin, PhD

Edward Bouwer, PhD

Guest Author: Bob Sheff, MD

Cover design by Kristine Rifkin

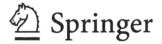 Springer

Erik Rifkin
Rifkin and Associates
10 E. Lee Street, #2107
Baltimore, MD 21202
USA

Edward Bouwer
Dept. of Geography & Environ. Engineering
Johns Hopkins University
3400 N. Charles Street
Baltimore, MD 21218
USA

ISBN: 978-0-387-48570-6 (hardcover)   ISBN: 978-0-387-48572-0 (eBook)
ISBN: 978-0-387-75165-8 (softcover)
DOI: 10.1007/978-0-387-48572-0
Springer New York Heidelberg Dordrecht London

Library of Congress Control Number: 2007921866

Printed on acid-free paper

Springer is part of Springer Science+Business Media (www.springer.com)

Advance Praise for *The Illusion of Certainty*

"This book does an excellent job of describing how health risks are calculated and how different ways of communicating these risks can dramatically change how people view these risks. The book is written in a way that most interested people can understand. The use of the Risk Characterization Theatre (RCT) is innovative and helps explain complex concepts in a simple, easy-to-understand fashion. The case studies are particularly informative and instructive."

– Gene Parkin, Professor, University of Iowa

"The Illusion of Certainty *is likely to make a few waves as it reaches the reading public. This would be an excellent and welcome outcome, as it is the unexamined conclusion that holds the greatest threat to well-being. By forcing the discussion of risk appraisal and the ways risk is presented to the public, Rifkin and Bouwer provide the discussion of risk with the counter-point that is necessary to its careful consideration."*

– Patricia Bender, Professor, Washburn University

"Even though I consider myself to be well-informed about health issues, their explanation of what they call 'the illusion of certainty' was a real eye-opener for me.... This book is 'must' reading, as patients and their families get more involved in making medical decisions and as citizens face critical questions about the environment."

– Bob Cooke, Writer, Creative Director, Cooke Communications

To Elaine

Still my best friend
after all these many years

E.R.

and

To Patricia

For her love, patience,
and understanding

E.J.B.

Foreword

Risk analysis and risk assessment have been with us long enough for the terms to sound familiar to most people. Standard fare for the nuclear power industry and the military for a half a century or more, risk assessment is now a routine aspect of environmental management, public health and individual medical decision making. There have been popular books on risk, and the current poker craze will likely spread risk concepts to an even wider (and younger) audience. Yet, despite all of this extensive and varied experience, we the analysts and practitioners have not done nearly enough to explain to the people who need to know what they need to know − especially the uncertainty inherent in risk estimates.

There are many instances in which the failure to communicate risk information accurately or completely has had an important and material impact on decisions and actions. I have been involved in some of these, ranging from local plans for water management to national decisions about nuclear waste. I have seen first hand the effects of poorly done risk assessments and bad risk communication, and especially the way in which the uncertainly of risk estimates is handled (or mishandled). The consequences of doing this wrong are high. It's high time that we addressed this gap in understanding, and this book is an excellent and important step in doing so.

There is nothing more effective than real stories, well-told, to engage readers, expose them to issues and help them to understand the complexity and subtlety of concepts. This book does just that, and it does it well. I doubt that anyone − especially a parent − will be able to put this book down after reading the first paragraph of Chapter 1.

I have known Erik Rifkin and Ed Bouwer for 25 years. These are two outstanding professionals and people, with broad and deep experience in risk assessment and its applications. They have been generous with that experience and knowledge, infusing this book with real cases – professional and personal – in which they've been involved. It makes for a compelling and rewarding experience for the reader.

Rifkin and Bouwer have also been courageous in writing this book. In going to the heart of what's been lacking in risk communication and management, they have taken on established thinking. As a result, this book may be controversial. In my view, a book like this is long overdue, and we all will be better for the reflection and debate it is likely to stimulate among scientists and policy-makers.

Jared L. Cohon, Ph.D.*
Pittsburgh, Pennsylvania
September, 2006

*President, Carnegie Mellon University

Preface

The use of risk assessment to characterize human health and ecological risks has become a well-accepted and widely-used practice throughout the world. The same principles are also used to evaluate the benefits from medical screening tests and drugs. Health benefit and risk portrayal has become a part of our everyday language and is frequently reported in the press, on TV, and on the radio. Here are some typical examples:

- Individuals living in a Pennsylvania town have a 1 in 100,000 increased risk of getting cancer due to the presence of arsenic in the drinking water.
- Chromium contamination in sediments significantly increases the risk of toxicity to fish and other aquatic organisms. Chromium is a known carcinogen.
- Evidence confirms that PCBs in the Hudson River have tripled the likelihood that certain species of fish will not be able to reproduce in 8 years.
- People with elevated blood serum cholesterol levels have a 100% greater risk of getting atherosclerosis and heart disease compared to individuals with normal cholesterol.
- Individuals taking statins to lower their blood serum cholesterol levels benefit by having fewer heart attacks.
- Research proves that smokers are 90% more likely to get lung cancer than individuals who have never smoked.
- Vioxx^{TM}, a COX-2 anti-inflammatory drug, has recently been withdrawn from all world markets. Researchers had found an increased risk of heart attack or stroke for people taking a standard dose for 18 months or more.
- People exposed to elevated radon levels in indoor air have a dramatically increased risk of getting lung cancer.

• Screening tests for prostate cancer (PSA) can determine which men are at a higher risk for getting this deadly disease.

Are these statements accurate? If so, are they meaningful? The above assertions mention just a few examples of the issues that many of us face. Individuals who are at risk for chronic ailments like heart disease take medicines and make dramatic lifestyle changes, hoping they will benefit. Corporations confronted with risks associated with the presence of environmental contaminants incur significant costs. Indeed, risk is an everyday reality, and it affects decisions we make in our lives. But where can we go for advice and guidance on decoding risk pronouncements?

Risk assessment is a valid and important scientific discipline, but the uncertainty in this process tends to be forgotten. Unfortunately, ignoring uncertainty has serious results: errors of interpretation, communication of misleading information, even dissemination of deceptive statements. The chance of a health benefit or risk can be reported as a relative number or an absolute number. It can be presented as a rate, a probability, or the cause of a positive or adverse effect. Since the use of risk assessment has become common-place, proper interpretation of health benefit and risk values is essential.

The purpose of this book is to provide individuals with the tools to interpret health benefit and risk values objectively, and to give the reader an understanding and appreciation of the risk assessment process. Included will be an explanation of the uncertainty inherent in the assessment of health benefits and risks, as well as an explanation of how communication and characterization can dramatically alter how those benefits and risks are perceived. Generally speaking, benefit and risk statements tend to be presented as if they were authoritative, definitive, and based on clear and unequivocal evidence. This leads to an illusion of certainty. In this context, this book compares and contrasts the differences between risk assessment and causality.

Case studies will be used to illustrate the strengths and limitations of characterizing certain health benefits and risks. Using the accepted risk assessment paradigm proposed by the National Research Council, these case studies will illustrate which benefit and risk values have merit and why other assessments fail to meet basic criteria.

This book was written and designed primarily to assist the public in comprehending and interpreting health benefit and risk information. It uses unique, visual presentations to explain the risks and benefits of medical screening tests and drugs, as well as the risks associated with exposure to environmental contaminants. This book should also be of interest to professionals in medicine, nursing, and public health. Government advisory and regulatory agencies, politicians, lawyers, engineers, and academicians should also find this book to be of value. In addition, this book could be used as supplemental information for a variety of undergraduate and graduate courses.

NOTICE: This book is intended as a reference guide on risk assessment, not as a medical guide to self-treatment. The information of a medical nature in this book is meant to help you make informed decisions about your health by providing a more careful and complete understanding of benefits, risks, and uncertainty. If you suspect you need medical treatment, you should discuss it with your primary care physician. If you are being treated for a medical condition or are on medication, do not change your treatment program without discussing it with your doctor.

Acknowledgments

We thank the many friends and colleagues who took the time to share with us their perspectives and knowledge about health benefits and risks and their experiences with risk assessment. We are grateful for their teachings and thoughts, which have assisted in nurturing this book.

We thank the following individuals for their participation in the review of portions of our manuscript: Patricia Bender, Washburn University; Karl Bourdeaux, Beveridge & Diamond, P.C.; Neal Durant, Geosyntec Consultants; Henry Honick, III, DDS; Joshua Klayman, University of Chicago; Gene Parkin, University of Iowa; Loren Regier, Saskatoon City Hospital; and an attorney who wishes to remain anonymous. We appreciate their candid and critical comments.

We were fortunate to have the expertise of Jessica Lawson, graduate student at Johns Hopkins University, who prepared our graphics, gathered information, assisted in editing the chapters, and worked with the publisher's specifications to produce the final document. In addition, she was instrumental in preparing the chapter on smoking. Many of the chapters were edited by Bob Cooke of Cooke Communications. We appreciate his efforts to make the writing more engaging and to clarify the presentation of the technical subjects.

Finally, special thanks to Jared Cohon, Carnegie Mellon University, for preparing a thoughtful Foreword to our book.

This book would not have been possible without the help of all of the individuals named above.

Contents

Part I: The Basics

Part II: Case Studies

Part III: Perspectives

Appendices

Abbreviations

AR	absolute risk
ARR	absolute risk reduction
AVS	acid volatile sulfides
CDC	Centers for Disease Control
CHD	coronary heart disease
COX-2	cyclooxygenase 2 enzyme
CRC	colorectal cancer
CVD	cardiovascular disease
CWA	Clean Water Act
DBPs	disinfection by-products
DRE	digital rectal examination
EPA	Environmental Protection Agency
ERA	ecological risk assessment
FDA	Food and Drug Administration
FOB	fecal occult blood
HAAs	haloacetic acids
HDL	high-density lipoprotein
HQ	hazard quotient
LC_{50}	inhaled lethal concentration at which 50% of the exposed population will die
LD_{50}	ingested lethal dose at which 50% of the exposed population will die
LDL	low-density lipoprotein
MCL	maximum contaminant level (in drinking water)
MDE	Maryland Department of the Environment
MRFIT	multiple risk factor intervention trial
MRI	magnetic resonance imaging
MSX	multinucleated sphere unknown

NAS   National Academy of Sciences
NCI   National Cancer Institute
NNT   number needed to treat
NOAA   National Oceanic and Atmospheric Administration
NOAEL   no observable adverse effect level
NRC   National Research Council
NSAIDs   non-steroidal anti-inflammatory drugs
PCBs   polychlorinated biphenyls
PSA   prostate-specific antigen
RCT   risk characterization theater
RfD   reference dose
RR   relative risk
RRR   relative risk reduction
TCE   trichloroethylene
THMs   trihalomethanes
VIGOR   Vioxx™ gastrointestinal outcomes research

Part I

The Basics

1. The Illusion of Certainty

When scientific uncertainty appears in public science settings, it could reduce the perceived authority of science.

Stephen C. Zehr[1]

We noticed the lump on the back of my seven-year-old son's calf, just below the knee, when he was lying on the living room rug watching television. At first we thought it was an insect bite or sting, but we couldn't find a red or elevated spot. Jason Rifkin was not in any pain and had absolutely no interest in my wife's suggestion that we take him to urgent care at the hospital "just to be sure."

The doctor who examined him wrote a referral to an orthopedic surgeon and suggested we make an appointment ASAP. At that point we became concerned, though we tried to maintain our composure in front of our son. It was Monday and the appointment wasn't until Thursday. I spent the next couple of days reviewing all the medical information I could find that seemed to relate to Jason's lump.

What struck me, more than anything else, was the uncertainty associated with diagnosing this condition. The range of possibilities was vast. It could have been a cyst (one of four or more types), a benign adipose tumor, a fatty deposit, a reaction to an infection – or it could have been a cancerous growth.

Each scientific article I read indicated that there were probabilities and risks of the lump being one thing or another. It became evident that it would be hard to predict or define, with any degree of certainty, the origin or nature of this lump. Nevertheless, I jotted down the possibilities and some notion of a risk level for each one. I thought we were now prepared to discuss the situation with the doctor, and I was relatively sure he would be able to explain the lump once he had a look at it. After all, he was an expert, a specialist, and came highly recommended.

The surgeon examined Jason and said that it was most likely a fluid-filled cyst, but without surgery he couldn't be sure. That was 27 years ago; today a noninvasive test, such as ultrasound or a magnetic resonance imaging (MRI) scan can help distinguish a simple cyst from other more serious possibilities. He ruled out any association with the bone but couldn't rule out cancer, and said the lump could cause problems if it continued to grow. In spite of all the uncertainty, he told us that the only reasonable option was surgery, and it should be scheduled ASAP. He took the time to answer all of my questions about options other than surgery and went on to say that surgical removal of the lump involved risks and potential complications, including permanent nerve damage.

We were about to say, "Go ahead, whatever you think best." After all, here was a trained medical practitioner giving us advice about one of the most important things in the world to us: the health of our son. How could we disagree? What did we know? But it just felt wrong. There were lingering questions about the insistence on surgery and who should make the decision.

In spite of all the uncertainty, the doctor's recommendation for surgery was unequivocal. He seemed to be convinced that this was the way to go. Or maybe he felt we needed the reassurance of a no-doubt-about-it response, as is the case with many patients. According to Dr. Atul Gawande, "The new orthodoxy about patient autonomy has a hard time acknowledging an awkward truth: patients frequently don't want the freedom that we've given them. That is, they're glad to have their autonomy respected, but the exercise of that autonomy means being able to relinquish it."[2]

You might assume that, in a case like ours, a physician recommending a course of action would base that decision on an understanding of tumors, as well as the physiology, morphology, and pathology of bones, nerves, muscles, tendons, and ligaments in my son's leg. In fact, his recommendation had little to do with any of these factors. Rather, it was based solely on his assessment of what type of intervention constituted an acceptable risk. A second or third medical opinion would most likely be based on the very same thing.

The need for surgery was far from being a clear-cut decision, like getting a shot of an antibiotic for a bacterial infection would have been. There were too many unanswered questions related to risks, too many basic issues which should have been raised. What was the probability that the lump was benign? What were the chances it was malignant? How did the cancer risks compare with the risks of surgery? Who should determine if a risk is acceptable? When there's a high level of uncertainty, as in our case, can an evidence-based decision be made? What is the risk in absolute terms? What is the risk in relative terms? What's the difference between the two?

The scientific literature was in agreement that this lump was most likely a benign cyst, which would disappear over time. But the real issue was the risk of cancer and how to weigh that against the risks of surgical complications.

Look at it this way: hypothetically,

- if we suppose that 1 out of every 1,000 operations results in permanent nerve damage,
- and that 1 out of every 1,000,000 lumps on children's legs turns out to be cancerous,
- then the risk of an adverse event is 1,000 times greater if you elect to have surgery.

This kind of information is critical for making an informed decision, but our orthopedic surgeon didn't seem to see it that way. At least he didn't see fit to share his views on this matter when we met with him. As a scientist, I couldn't figure out why not.

Without really thinking, I asked the surgeon, "What would you do if your son had the same condition?"

He stared back at me for a moment, unable to answer. His hesitation gave me the confidence to say, "We've decided not to opt for surgery. The risk of complications is too great. Based on our research, we think it's probably a cyst and, in all probability, it will disappear."

The surgeon was taken aback and told us in no uncertain terms that this was not our decision to make. He would have the final say in this matter. When we respectfully disagreed, he went on to advise us that we would be solely responsible if complications arose as a result of our decision. I thanked him for his time, and Jason, my wife, and I went home.

For months after that day in the doctor's office, I had sleepless nights, misgivings about our decision, contentious discussions with my wife, and anxiety about the potential consequences of our choice.

The Growing Reliance on Risk Assessment

For many health problems, the decision on how to deal with them is a simple one. There's a reassuringly high level of certainty, made possible by major advances in medicine and in our understanding of the impacts of exposure to environmental contaminants. For many serious diseases, the causative agents have been clearly identified and then either contained or eradicated. Books such as Rachel Carson's *Silent Spring*[3] increased public awareness of the human health and ecological risks from contaminants in air, water, soil, and sediments. This awareness led to the passage of long-overdue legislation and regulations designed to protect public health and the environment.

As medical and environmental health concerns were addressed and major discoveries allowed us to reduce illness and improve the health of ecosystems, expectations became very high. The public, as well as politicians, anticipated continued success. But science couldn't keep up with the expectations. The search to find cures and to improve environmental quality gained momentum, but as the focus turned to chronic debilitating diseases such as heart disease, cancer, and diabetes, and to the effects of low levels of environmental contaminants like dioxin and PCBs, the results were less clear. These were murkier waters. Precise cause and effect relationships were not evident. Unverified theoretical models, rather than direct observation, were used to evaluate problems. In short, the level of uncertainty was rising, and it was severely limiting our ability to make confident decisions regarding health issues.

The scientific, regulatory, and medical communities have been forced to turn to an analytical technique known as risk assessment for answers.

When cause and effect cannot be delineated clearly, risk assessment is a way to navigate in this "iffier" territory.

The concept of risk is easy to understand. It is, simply, a possibility. Not a sure thing, not a certainty, but something that might happen or bring about some result. High probability equates to high predictability and makes an event more likely. Low probability equates to low predictability and makes an event less likely. But high or low or anywhere in between, the outcome is uncertain.

From the start, this uncertainty inherent in the risk assessment process has been problematic. Risk assessment specialists pointed out that, when discussing risks, doctors and other authorities needed to explain uncertainty to patients and communities. Unfortunately, this has rarely happened. The reasons are manifold, but probably relate to our need for answers. Uncertainty causes anxiety, particularly when it involves our health. Environmental scientists, physicians, and drug companies try to respond by giving us what we want, but the uncertainty often gets lost in the process.

The public has not been properly educated and informed about uncertainty, so when medical or environmental options are presented, people are not equipped to make evidence-based decisions. Today, we are in a position where millions of us are being asked to accept medical procedures and environmental management practices which are in fact based on uncertain scientific findings. And while they may come recommended by the authorities, these recommendations reflect someone else's determination of what risk is acceptable or unacceptable for us. In effect, decisions are made for us. What's more, those decisions are often less fact-based than we are led to believe.

This is not an outright condemnation; risk assessment is a valid and important scientific discipline. But the uncertainty in the process tends to be ignored. As a result, errors of interpretation are common, and the dissemination of misleading or even deceptive information is widespread. The chance of a health benefit or risk continues to be reported using terms with specific meanings that few people really understand, such as relative numbers, absolute numbers, rates, risk factors, death benefits, probabilities, and cause and effect. And as more emphasis is placed on chronic debilitating diseases without clearly defined causes, these descriptions of health benefits and risks – undefined and without complete documentation or even sufficient supporting evidence – will appear more and more frequently in coming years.

Since risk assessment is becoming so commonplace, it is essential to learn how to interpret health benefit and risk values properly. Though we may often shy away from making decisions about our health or the environment, we really do need to understand risk and uncertainty so that we can address these difficult issues.

About six months after our meeting with the orthopedic surgeon, my wife and I were startled by a cry from the backyard, where Jason was playing with a couple of friends. One of them had accidentally landed on his leg, the one with the lump. The bad news was that it hurt. The good news was that the lump was gone. It was, indeed, a harmless Baker's cyst which had broken and released its fluid.

When we saw the doctor one last time, he acknowledged that my wife and I had made the right decision. However, he added that if he were confronted with the same situation in the future, he would recommend surgery again. I suggested that an objective discussion about risk factors and acceptable risk would be helpful. He thanked me for my views.

What are the Real Risks of Dioxin?

The phone call was from Spencer, a colleague who was the CEO of a department store chain headquartered in the Midwest, and he sounded a bit frantic. He had just read an article in the local newspaper about airborne dioxin releases from a nearby waste recovery facility. The state regulatory agency had assessed the situation. The risks, according to the article, were 200% higher than the Environmental Protection Agency's (EPA) acceptable limit for this cancer-causing contaminant. He was concerned about how the release of this carcinogen might affect his son. Since birth, his two-year-old boy had been beset with breathing problems and seemed more prone to illness than most. Spencer's question to me was, "What does this mean, and what can I do about it?"

I explained that the EPA had established acceptable risk levels for carcinogenic contaminants. These levels were not based on science, but rather on value judgments by the EPA regarding what constitutes an appropriate level of risk for exposed populations throughout the country. The EPA's acceptable risk levels were usually adopted by state regulatory agencies. The philosophy was to err on the side of safety. Therefore, acceptable risk levels, particularly for carcinogens, tended to be quite conservative, set low to ensure that they were protective of human health. I also pointed out that the inherent uncertainty in the risk assessment process should be considered before putting too much stock in any newspaper article.

In most instances, the acceptable risk level for substances like dioxin that are known to cause cancer in humans is one additional cancer for every million individuals over a lifetime of exposure. (Technically, there is no such thing as zero risk as long as a single molecule of a contaminant can be detected.) By this definition, a risk of two in a million (commonly expressed as 2/1,000,000) is unacceptable.

Spencer was confused. There weren't even a million people in his city, he said, so wouldn't the acceptable level of exposure impact less than one individual? I told him he was correct. As it turns out, a one in a million risk would mean that approximately 300 additional lifetime cancers would occur throughout the country if everyone in the nation were exposed to the particular chemical. While the EPA has to evaluate risk for the entire US population, I told my friend that he would be well-advised to stay focused on the increased risk to his son.

Spencer had more questions. Isn't dioxin one of the most potent carcinogens known to man? The answer was yes. However, this high toxicity had already been accounted for in the risk number reported in the newspaper. Risk levels incorporate factors such as relative toxicity and adjust acceptable exposures accordingly. For dioxin, due to its high toxicity, exposure levels are set to parts per quadrillion. For other less toxic contaminants, you can be exposed to a much higher level (parts per million, billion, or trillion) and still have the same acceptable one in a million risk.

Frustrated, my colleague asked, "But how does all that relate to my son?" I then explained how health risk assessments, both medical and environmental, use relative risks – like the 200% figure in the article Spencer read – which almost always distort the picture.

Environmental regulatory agencies use relative risks to accentuate the adverse effects of exposure to environmental contaminants, which is consistent with their mandate to err on the side of protection.

On the other hand, pharmaceutical companies use relative numbers to describe the benefits of drugs. Why? One of the objectives of the pharmaceutical industry is to sell more drugs, and the benefits of those drugs tend to sound more impressive when relative numbers are used.

Furthermore, relative risks are almost always used in news reports relating to health risks, perhaps because they result in more sensational stories that boost ratings or newspaper sales.

In all these cases, it would be wise to consider the source and be mindful of the agenda of any group that's communicating about risk. The discussion and understanding of absolute risk, relative risk, and uncertainty are essential to objective decision-making. With this in mind, Spencer and I turned to the subject of dioxin.

Dioxin is formed as an unwanted by-product when organic chemicals and chlorine are subjected to high temperatures in waste recovery facilities, pulp mills, and factories that produce PVC plastic and chlorinated herbicides. Improper releases can result in contamination near these sources, such as downstream from pulp mills and in soil. Contamination has forced the relocation of families from communities like Times Beach and Love Canal.

Exposure to certain levels of dioxin causes a wide range of effects including cancer, changes to the nervous system, reduced immunity, skin disfigurement, and modifications to the DNA in the nucleus of our cells. Scientists studying dioxin believe that health effects will occur at the part per trillion level in body fat. Unfortunately, dioxin is very resistant to degradation; it settles on crops and contaminates lakes, streams, and the ocean. Spencer then repeated his question, "How does all of this relate to my son?"

I suggested we start with relative risk. If 1/1,000,000 is his state's acceptable level of risk for carcinogens, then 3/1,000,000 is expressed as a relative risk of 200%. That's because relative risk is a comparison of the numerators in the two fractions, and 3 is 200% greater than 1.

We then turned to absolute risk, which is a much more appropriate and meaningful way to measure health risks for individuals like Spencer's son. Using the same dioxin numbers, the absolute increase in risk would be 0.0002% (see Chap. 2 for how to calculate absolute risk) – not a very significant difference. So even though dioxin is very toxic, exposure levels were low enough in Spencer's city that the rate of increase in health effects would be miniscule. What's more, as I explained to Spencer, the uncertainty in the EPA's risk assessment was very high. As a matter of fact, the dioxin release might not increase the risk of cancer at all. According to the EPA cancer guidelines document, there is an equal probability that the risk is zero.

Finally, I referred to an article in Science magazine written by William Ruckelshaus and published in 1983.[4] The former EPA Administrator discussed how risk assessment suffers from fundamental uncertainties:

- The actual mechanisms that cause cancer and other hazards are largely unknown
- It is difficult to extrapolate what might happen at very low doses from an experiment that only examines the effects of relatively high doses
- Humans may not be affected in the same way as test animals are
- It is not always practical or possible for experiments to determine latent effects and latency periods
- Some individuals will be more sensitive to adverse effects, while others will be more resistant
- Exposure to more than one substance at once could have synergistic or co-carcinogenic effects
- It is hard to assess past and present exposure levels and dispersion patterns for contaminants

In short, he asserted that there are uncertainties in virtually every area of required knowledge.[4] More than twenty years later, the situation remains essentially the same.

Spencer wondered why this kind of information isn't communicated by the state and federal agencies regarding health risks. He wondered why the local journalists weren't more rigorous in their reporting. He wondered, most of all, how people throughout the country could be expected to make health decisions based on unverified assumptions and an unacceptably high degree of uncertainty.

The Illusion of Certainty

Risk assessment is a relatively new and evolving scientific tool. While risk analysis can be used to make general predictions regarding health risks and risk factors, we must always be aware of its limitations. Risk numbers are, by definition, uncertain and based on value-laden assumptions and ambiguous models. Unlike accurate predictions in the physical sciences, risk values commonly vary by orders of magnitude, i.e., factors of ten, and are misleading if the uncertainty associated with them is not made clear. The perception is that the benefits of a medical action or an environmental cleanup are known with certainty. For various reasons, discussed in this book, this is not always the case.

Medical health and environmental health risk assessments are conducted by different groups and institutions that use different formats and methods to communicate about risk. With few exceptions, attempts to have these groups work together have been unsuccessful. Currently, if the health risks are associated with cholesterol levels, smoking, or the presence of prostate proteins in the blood, then risk analysis is assumed to be under the jurisdiction of the medical community. If, on the other hand, health risk concerns relate to cancer, non-cancer effects, or ecological risks from exposure to contaminants, then the EPA and state regulatory agencies are the primary sources of advice and guidance. Unfortunately, although both of these groups apply similar risk assessment principles for assessing health risks, neither of them systematically includes an explanation of the uncertainty in their evaluation of risks, and neither provides a clear explanation of relative and absolute risks.

The purpose of this book is to provide the reader with an understanding and appreciation of the risk assessment process, the ability to interpret health benefit and risk values objectively, and the means to use this information in making critical decisions regarding health risk factors. All too often, health benefit and risk statements are presented as if they were authoritative, definitive, and based on clear and compelling evidence. The result is what we call the *illusion of certainty.*

Roadmap

A brief roadmap for this book is provided here to guide the reader through the content and organization of the topics. The first part (Chaps. 1-5) focuses on background information, on the process of how health benefits and risks are characterized, and on the associated uncertainty. Examples demonstrating the benefits from mammograms and the risks from dioxin exposure appear in Part One.

The first few chapters set the stage for the second part, containing the essence or "meat" of the book: case studies that clearly summarize the health benefits and risks associated with medical screening tests, drugs, and environmental contaminants. In these chapters, an innovative and straight-forward visual aid is used to demonstrate the benefits from pro-state and colon cancer screening and statins, as well as the risks from smoking, elevated cholesterol, Vioxx^{TM}, chlorinated drinking water, and radon. Part Two also contains chapters on the uncertainty inherent in ecological risk assessment, with Asian oysters and chromium as examples. The authors have first-hand experience with many of the issues and situations presented in these case studies.

The third part concludes the book with two perspectives on how risk assessment is relevant in our everyday lives. The first of these chapters is by guest author Bob Sheff, MD. Dr. Sheff is a radiologist and was an administrator for one of the largest medical managed-care systems in the United States. His chapter emphasizes why it is critically important for patients to develop an understanding of how health benefits and risks are characterized and communicated.

Certain sections within the first few chapters describe theory and terminology, and may take a little longer to grasp than the more visual case studies. While these sections are not essential to the practical examples, they do lay the foundation for understanding the origin of the data and concepts in the case studies, which may be read in any order. Even if you do not read this book from cover to cover, we believe you will find the discussion in the final two chapters particularly informative.

2. Cause and Effect vs. Risk Factors

Risk estimates are even more important in evaluating screening and preventive care, since individuals are counseled to seek these services. For this counsel to be ethical, not only must the action not be harmful, but it must have a reasonable chance of benefiting the person.

Lester B. Lave[1]

Alice went to see her doctor for her annual physical. Noting that Alice was now in her forties, her doctor recommended that she get a mammogram. But Alice said she wasn't sure she wanted to do that. She had read that some experts questioned whether the benefits of the procedure were worth the inconvenience, discomfort, costs, and potential adverse effects from intervention, like radiation or biopsies. Before making a decision, she wanted more information. Only in the best of all possible worlds would Alice's doctor take the time to discuss all of these issues fully, but let's assume she did.

She told Alice that a mammogram is only a screening test designed to detect abnormalities – lumps – in the breast. She explained that if a lump were found, further testing might be necessary to see if it correlated to breast cancer. The presence of a lump would not mean that she had breast cancer, just that additional procedures might be required. In other words, there is no cause and effect relationship because the presence of a lump in the breast is not *always* associated with cancer.

Seeing that Alice was listening intently, this exemplary doctor continued.

Cause and Effect

The doctor explained that when there are two events, with the first consistently resulting in the second, scientists recognize them as cause and effect. The cause makes something happen. The effect is what happens. She gave Alice some medical examples:

- HIV is the cause, AIDS is the effect.
- The polio virus is the cause, poliomyelitis is the effect.
- A type of parasite called a plasmodium is the cause, malaria is the effect.

In these instances, medical science has demonstrated with a high degree of certainty that a disease will occur if the agent known to be causative is present. *By definition of cause and effect, the disease-causing agent must always be present if the effect is to occur.* When a specific cause is consistently linked with a specific effect, there's little uncertainty about the diagnosis, and intervention is almost always warranted.

A number of cause and effect relationships have been confirmed. The presence of adequate levels of certain environmental contaminants (like asbestos) or specific infectious agents (such as bacteria or viruses) has been directly linked to specific diseases or health effects. Unfortunately, that's not the case with many chronic conditions, including cancer.

Establishing causality for cancer is problematic because cancer doesn't appear immediately after exposure to a cancer-causing substance. It seems to require a latency period, and this delay makes it harder – and often simply impossible – to figure out what caused it.

One typical determinant for causality is exposure to an environmental insult, like a carcinogen. As exposure to the carcinogen increases, the incidence of the disease usually increases as well. But if we can't quantify exposure, it is difficult to determine the relationship between exposure and disease with any degree of accuracy. We often find ourselves in this situation when dealing with environmental exposures because relevant levels of contaminants are very low. In most cases, is it virtually impossible to determine the time and degree of initial and subsequent exposures.

Scientists are more likely to conclude that a particular agent causes a particular form of cancer if it can be demonstrated in epidemiological studies, which are large, controlled studies of people. But with a few exceptions – asbestos exposure causing mesothelioma or radon exposure causing lung cancer in miners, for example – we have not yet been able to correlate exposure to potential carcinogens with specific types of cancer. Without multiple studies showing consistent results that verify causality, uncertainty remains. Animal experiments are another commonly used approach for determining whether or not exposure to a substance will result in cancer. Results from these experiments are used in mathematical models to predict the level of exposure which might cause cancer in humans, but they often rely on unverified, controversial assumptions that leave us with a high level of uncertainty.

Risk Factors

If a direct cause and effect relationship cannot be demonstrated between a disease and an agent or substance that is present, yet there seems to be a statistical association between the two, the agent suspected of being asso-ciated with an effect is called a *risk factor*. In other words, *a risk factor is a biological condition, substance, or behavior that has an association with but has not been proven to cause an event or disease.*

With health problems like coronary heart disease, cancer, stroke, and diabetes – which typically have long latency periods and no documented causative agent – the medical community uses a risk factor approach to determine intervention strategies. Yet there is considerable inherent uncer-tainty when risk factors and risk analysis are part of the equation. Due to this uncertainty, we should avoid equating "risk factor" and "cause." They're simply not the same. Consider these examples: elevated choles-terol is termed a risk factor but not the cause of coronary heart disease; a lump detected in breast tissue is a risk factor but not the cause of breast cancer; childhood obesity is a risk factor but not the cause of diabetes. This distinction is critically important, since it can be very difficult to prove a statistically significant relationship between a risk factor and an effect.

Identifying a risk factor is valuable only to the extent that it can be used to predict an increased frequency or probability that a particular event or disease will occur. So when Alice was told that a lump would be classified a risk factor, it meant that a lump in the breast may or may not be associated with cancer. Her doctor explained that lumps are not necessarily cancerous.

It was becoming clear to Alice that asking the right questions and being able to interpret the answers was going to be essential if she was going to make an informed decision about having a mammogram. She needed to know:

- How strong is the association between the presence of a lump and cancer?
- Can that association be used to predict an increased frequency or probability of breast cancer?
- What is the uncertainty in the studies that have been conducted?
- Are the benefits of a mammogram worth the time, money, and potential negative impacts from intervention?
- What about the risks associated with radiation from mammograms?
- Why are risks characterized by some as significant and by others as trivial?

Ordinarily, people don't ask questions like these. But they should, since the answers leave room for people to reach different conclusions, based on how they feel about taking risks. Understanding uncertainty and the way health risks are presented is critical to making an informed decision.

Alice was fortunate that her doctor believed in the patient's right to be part of the decision-making process, understood risk analysis, and was willing to take the time to explain the basic concepts and answer all her questions. The physician proceeded to explain that the widespread use of mammograms is designed to reduce the risks and, therefore, the death rates from cancer. But, she continued, there is a great deal of controversy surrounding the benefits of mammograms. In fact, a well documented report published in the year 2000 by two Danish scientists questioned the appropriateness of conducting this screening test without first identifying the actual benefits and predicted risks.[2]

The public hears about health benefits and risks from many sources, and there are a number of different ways to talk about their significance. While all of these approaches may be scientifically legitimate, the misinterpretation of some of the statistical relationships involved can lead to inappropriate medical intervention.

Alice wasn't a scientist, and she knew virtually nothing about statistics. Was the subject about to get too technical for her to follow? Her doctor's encouragement at this point makes sense for everyone:

It may get a little complicated, but in a relatively short time you will be able to master what you need to know to make an informed decision. Given the importance of this matter, it's worth the effort.

Absolute Risk versus Relative Risk

As Alice's doctor told her, if you understand the concepts of relative risk and absolute risk, and nothing else, you'll be amazed at your newfound ability to interpret newspaper articles and TV reports on drug and diet benefits, risks, and the value of screening tests like mammograms.

Absolute risk is *your* risk of developing a disease over a specified period of time. Absolute risk is generally calculated for chronic diseases and can be expressed in different ways. For example, if it has been determined that 1 person in a 100 will get a disease, this can be expressed as a 1% absolute risk, a 0.01 absolute risk, or a 1 in 100 absolute risk.

Absolute risk reduction (ARR) is the difference between the absolute risks in two groups. One way of expressing the ARR is as a percentage death rate. For example, ARR could refer to differences in breast cancer death rates between two groups of women: those who get and those who don't get mammograms over a period of time (typically in the range of five to fifteen years).

Unfortunately, *absolute* risk and ARR values are rarely provided to the public. Instead, when we hear about health risks or risk reduction, we're actually hearing *relative* numbers. *Relative risk reduction* (RRR) uses the ratio of two absolute risk numbers to measure how much the risk is reduced in one group compared to another group. With RRR numbers, the absolute risk levels for the two groups are not communicated. This is a serious problem, because relative and absolute numbers can give very different impressions, and you must have absolute risk information in order to make an informed decision.

Calculating relative risks and the relative risk reduction (RRR) is a valid statistical method, but it tends to distort the benefits to individuals when it is used to explain health risks. The real benefit is usually much smaller than it may appear. The benefits of screening tests, including mammograms, are almost always presented in relative terms. The RRR approach may be helpful to scientists and public health officials, but patients are not really among the beneficiaries. Since RRR is used by drug companies, the media, physicians, and others to characterize health risks, it's important to understand how it differs from *absolute* risk. Hopefully, the following hypothetical examples will make this clear.

A Hypothetical 5-Year Diabetes Drug Study

- A hypothetical study investigated the effectiveness of a drug in reducing deaths from complications due to the onset of diabetes. The study group consisted of twenty thousand men, all of whom had diabetes.
- Ten thousand men were given the drug and the other ten thousand were given a placebo. The study went on for five years.
- By the end of the 5-year study, one individual in the experimental group (given the drug) had died of diabetes. In the control (placebo) group, two individuals died of diabetes.
- The absolute risk reduction (ARR), in terms of the percentage death rate, is the difference in death rates for the two groups. For the group given the drug, the death rate was 0.01% (because 1/10,000 = 0.01%). For the control group, it was 2/10,000 (because 2/10,000 = 0.02%). When you subtract 0.01% from 0.02%, the answer is 0.01%. So the ARR is 0.01%.

- Another way to look at these results is to say that of 10,000 diabetics in a room, only one would benefit from receiving this drug over a 5-year period.

Unlike absolute risks, relative risks and RRR are, by far, the most common and widely used methods for characterizing health risks. These are the values you hear and see in the media. In this example of a diabetes drug study, this would mean comparing the number of individuals who died in each of the two groups. To calculate relative risk reduction you would compare the 2 in 2/10,000 and the 1 in 1/10,000. The reduction is from 2 to 1; there is one fewer death in the group receiving the drug. Since this difference of 1 death is 50% of the 2 deaths observed in the control group, *the relative risk reduction or RRR is 50%.*

Same study. Same actual results. Expressed as 0.01% ARR or as 50% RRR. Quite a difference! Being told that taking a drug will halve your chance of dying sounds much better than being told that taking a drug would change the death rate by 0.01%, or that one person out of 10,000 would benefit over a 5-year period!

To make her point about the problem even clearer, Alice's doctor posed a variation on this hypothetical case. What if the drug was used to treat a rare disease rather than diabetes? Assume the death rate without the drug is 2 out of 1,000,000 and with the drug is 1 out of 1,000,000. *The absolute percentage rate difference is now 0.0001%, but the relative risk reduction is still 50%.* The calculation of this RRR is statistically valid, but the chance of benefiting from the drug is literally one in a million!

The Number Needed to Treat

Alice understood everything so far and was ready for the next technical term: *the number needed to treat* (NNT). This term is used frequently in the medical literature and refers to the number of people who need to be treated in order for one person to benefit.

Let's suppose that 4 out of 100 people will normally become victims of a particular disease. A pharmaceutical company reports that a new drug reduces the relative risk of getting the disease by 25%. This means that of the original 4 victims, one will be spared if all 100 take the new drug (25% of 4 = 1).

Here is another way to look at the situation: on average, in a group of 100 people who don't take the drug, 4 will get the disease. In a group of 100 people who do take the drug, only 3 people will get the disease. *Therefore, 100 people need to take the treatment for 1 person to benefit. The NNT is 100.*

How to Characterize Risks

After hearing these examples, Alice wanted to apply her new knowledge and determine if mammograms would be appropriate for her. She still wanted advice and guidance from her physician, but she now realized that she would need to make the final decision based on her own perception of acceptable risk. Her doctor cautioned that before making this decision she needed to learn more about uncertainty and the different ways to characterize, or define, risks. The lesson continued.

Let's say a man reads a report from one of the major wire services in his local newspaper indicating that a new drug reduces the risk of getting heart disease by 50%. Since his father had heart disease as a relatively young man and he is overweight, he's tempted to buy and take these pills. His wife suggests he investigate the claims of risk reduction a little more closely.

The study group consisted of 1,000 men who received the drug and another 1,000 men who didn't receive any treatment. In the group receiving the treatment, two individuals were diagnosed with heart disease during the eight-year study. In the control group, four individuals got heart disease. This represented a 50% RRR (2 is 50% of 4; compare the treated group to the control group) and a 0.2% ARR (4/1,000 = an absolute risk of 0.4%; 2/1,000 = 0.2%; 0.4% minus 0.2% = 0.2%). As is often the case, the drug company only advertised the RRR of 50%. According to the study, there were also a number of serious side effects associated with taking the drug that included possible liver damage, muscular problems, and impotence.

He can't find any written information presenting the risks and benefits in a meaningful way that would help him make his decision. He realizes that the payments for this drug will be a burden. What should he do?

He decides to ignore the RRR value and focus on absolute risks instead. With his doctor's help, he finds out that there is a 3 in 1,000 chance of developing serious side effects (which are often termed "contraindications" on prescription labels). Therefore, while the risk of getting heart disease would be decreased to 0.2%, the risk of serious complications would be 0.3%. A heart attack could be fatal. The side effects would be less likely to be fatal. He also has to factor in the prohibitively high cost of the drug. It's a tough decision, but at least he has a factual basis for making an informed choice. When patients understand the real potential benefits of a drug or a procedure, they may be better able to decide if it is appropriate to forgo a treatment that may not only be expensive but also have unwanted or dangerous side effects.

Returning to the subject of Alice's mammogram, her doctor referred back to the Danish study in 2000. Its authors found essentially no meaningful decrease in breast cancer deaths in Sweden, where mammograms to screen women for breast cancer had been recommended since 1985. Furthermore, their article stated that "screening for breast cancer with mammography is unjustified."[2]

This statement was based on results from 129,750 women who had mammograms in the late 1970s and early 1980s and a comparison group of 117,260 women who did not have mammograms. Death rates from breast cancer were calculated over a twelve-year period. The death rate for the group that had mammograms was 0.4% (511 died of breast cancer) and for the control group, 0.5% (584 breast cancer deaths). The ARR is the difference between 0.5% and 0.4%, or 0.1%. This meant that 1,000 women would have to get mammograms biennially for twelve years in order to prevent one single death from breast cancer. It was on this basis that the authors recommended that mammography screening was not justified.[2]

In light of this information, Alice wanted to know why mammograms are routinely recommended to millions of women every year. Her physician explained that there have been numerous articles in the last five years on both sides of the issue, some agreeing with the Danish scientists and others refuting their findings. Many scientists questioned bias in the studies selected for their analysis, and others questioned the experimental design of the analysis itself. On the other hand, equally prominent scientists have fully concurred with the finding that mammograms are not warranted.

Much of the controversy centered on the characterization of risk. Alice's physician asked her to use her new knowledge to calculate the RRR, using data reported in the study. Alice had learned her lesson well. She said that the difference between 0.5% and 0.4% was 0.1%; and that 0.1 was 20% of 0.5. Therefore, the RRR demonstrated a 20% relative death benefit among women who have had mammograms. The difference between a 20% RRR and a 0.1% ARR sounded dramatic, even though both numbers described the same information.

Using exactly the same data set, Fig. 2.1 demonstrates the rather striking differences in characterizing risk when using RRR and ARR. Using RRR, patients would be told that women who have biennial mammograms are 20% less likely to die of breast cancer. Using ARR, a patient would learn that there is a 0.1% reduction in the breast cancer death rate for women who have biennial mammograms, and that the NNT is 1,000. When event rates are low, ARR becomes smaller. RRR often remains constant. This is yet another reason to question the value of relative risks.

Her doctor then cited another case, which involved the characterization of risks and benefits from taking the drug tamoxifen. News headlines like "Tamoxifen Cuts Breast Cancer Risk by 50% in Healthy Women!" were proclaiming the drug. Of course, the media reported the RRR. In the actual medical study, less than 2% of women taking tamoxifen got breast cancer, and less than 3% of those taking the placebo got breast cancer. The absolute rate difference was about 1%.[3]

Alice now understood how important it was to know the absolute risk values when making a decision based on risk analysis. But she wondered if there were other factors to consider on the risk side of the equation. What about radiation risks, or risks from associated procedures like biopsies? What about the uncertainty in the large studies that served as the basis for the characterization of risk?

A. Absolute Risk Reduction

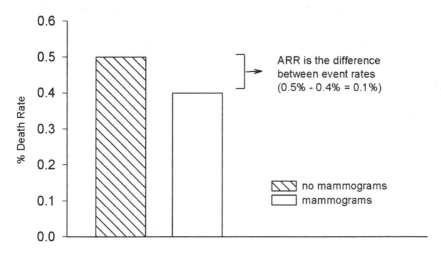

B. Relative Risk Reduction

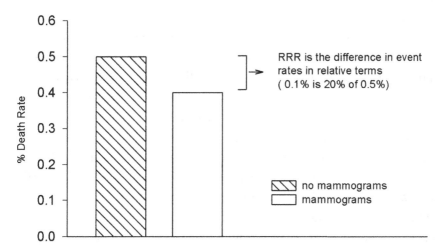

Fig. 2.1. The bars in both graphs represent the percent death rate for women in Swedish mammography trials. It is obvious that graphs A and B represent the same data, which are used to calculate both absolute risk reduction and relative risk reduction. **A.** Absolute Risk Reduction (ARR) is 0.1%, **B.** Relative Risk Reduction (RRR) is 20%

Alice's doctor told her that her questions were well-founded, but that she was not aware of any report combining all of these factors to determine overall risks from mammograms.

Radiation from repeated mammograms is a real concern. Although dosage levels have been reduced thanks to modern equipment, screening at an early age and frequent examinations would increase radiation dosage and, perhaps, the chance of cancer. Whether that increased chance would meaningfully impact the ARR is unclear.

Her doctor then addressed Alice's question on associated and potentially unnecessary procedures. Doctors will order a number of "additional tests" for every 10,000 mammograms given to healthy women. These include 358 breast examinations by ultrasound, 104 "aspiration" biopsies (where fluid and cells from the area of the breast with the abnormality are removed), and 209 surgical biopsies (removal of part of the breast containing the abnormality). As it turns out, the majority of the "abnormal" mammograms will prove to be false positives, and only about 25 of the women will have breast cancer.[4] The bottom line was that the risks from these procedures didn't seem to be reflected in the ARR either.

The doctor thought that Alice's point about uncertainty in the large epidemiological studies of hundreds of thousands of women was a very important one and merited some additional discussion. While it is generally agreed that there is less uncertainty when studies involve people rather than animals, there are still many areas that can be problematic. Were there enough people in the control and experimental groups? Was the analysis conducted in a rigorous manner? Was there an appropriate statistical evaluation of the data? Was there a description of the statistical methods used? Was bias identified and addressed properly? And so forth.

The design of the study, how it is conducted, how the results are interpreted – these are all areas of potential uncertainty. Without a description and explanation of this uncertainty, it's difficult to characterize absolute risks accurately.

Risk characterization is designed to bridge the gaps between doing a risk assessment, choosing risk control options such as medical intervention, and determining acceptable risk, i.e., risk management. Theoretically, risk characterization describes the risks both to individuals and to populations, communicates the results of the risk assessment, develops clear and implicit statements of strengths and weaknesses, and evaluates the overall quality of the assessment. In characterizing health risks, care must be taken not to trivialize or exaggerate risks. Perhaps most important, the objective characterization of risk requires that numerical estimates never be separated from the descriptive information about uncertainty, because numbers tend to take on a life of their own.

We want to believe that diagnostic tests *must* be beneficial. But this view does not always properly weigh the merits of a test against other factors, such as side effects and the consequences of false positive results. Deciding what level of risk is acceptable should involve a value judgment on the part of the patient.

Alice now understood what she really needed to make an informed decision, so she asked her doctor for objective, written information including charts, which would compare individual and population risks and discuss absolute risks, absolute risk reduction, decreased life expectancy, risks from intervention, uncertainty, and overall benefits from mammography. Apologetically, the doctor said she didn't know where to locate that information and doubted whether it could be found in any one place. It was clear to both Alice and her doctor that it would be extremely helpful if health risk assessments – including a full and open discussion of uncertainty – were made transparent to the public. Such information would lead to more appropriate use of screening tests and a greater understanding of drug benefits and side effects.

Alice decided to postpone any decision on having a mammogram until she could track down, review, and interpret all the relevant information. Her doctor agreed.

Summary

It has been estimated that 30 million mammograms are done in the US each year. During the past five years, there have been dozens of articles in reputable, peer-reviewed medical journals addressing the central question: is screening for breast cancer with mammograms justifiable? There are many different views on the subject, but one thing is clear – it is a controversial issue.

It is likely that a large percentage of women will be satisfied to take the recommendation of their physicians and continue to have annual or biennial mammograms. It is also reasonable to assume that many women would want to know more about the risks and benefits of mammography before making a decision about having the test. Unfortunately, at present patients are not given the information they need to make an informed choice. And in most cases they don't even know what they're missing. Risks and benefits associated with screening tests and medical intervention in general are almost always characterized in terms of RRR. As a result, reports in the popular media, medical literature, and pharmaceutical advertisements often make the benefits seem far more impressive than they really are.

While RRR is a useful yardstick for research scientists, it should not be used by the public to assess the risks and benefits of screening tests. Far more weight should be given to ARR values.

ARR is the simple difference between event rates, such as death rates. If the reduction in absolute risk is communicated, patients can easily determine the number of individuals who would have to be screened for one person to benefit, known as the number needed to treat (NNT). This may well be the most meaningful reference point for patients interested in being involved in the decision-making process. RRR values do not provide any insight into this very important measure of risk.

In the case of mammograms, the absolute risk reduction is 0.1%, which means that the NNT is 1,000. Using ARR, patients would be told that there is a 0.1% reduction in deaths among women who have biennial mammograms when compared to those who have not had biennial mammograms. Therefore, 1,000 mammograms would have to be given in order for one person to benefit.

Additional information on other risks from intervention, including biopsies, radiation, false positives, and false negatives should also be provided to women who are facing a decision on whether or not to have mammograms. A woman would then be in position to consider all the risks and weigh the odds that she would be the one individual in 1,000 to benefit from biennial mammograms. Would she make the same decision if the NNT were 100,000? What if it were 10? The decision would be personal, and it would depend on how risk-averse that woman was. What's right for one woman might not be right for another.

In light of this situation, the medical community should provide women with an accurate assessment of the harm and benefits from screening mammography, even if this means acknowledging the overall uncertainty in assessing this health risk. Different individuals may well prefer different options when it comes to choosing a treatment based on a risk assessment.

Given the large numbers of women who might welcome and benefit from this kind of educational material, it is difficult to understand why it is not already being provided routinely. Whatever the reason, it leaves women today with two choices: go along with the status quo, or demand objective information from their doctors regarding the risks, benefits, and uncertainty associated with mammograms.

3. Reframing the Debate

First of all, the obvious should be stated. For scientists, science communication with a lay audience is almost always a secondary issue.

Christine Russell[1]

The general public is faced with a difficult and perhaps even insurmountable task: find and decipher objective information about health benefits and risks in order to make the right decisions about medical and environmental issues.

Why is it so hard? Because, although there are plenty of articles and reports advising people to learn about uncertainty and the differences between absolute and relative risks, there's virtually nothing giving examples of *exactly what should be done*. The complex technical information is not translated into a straightforward, simple format that presents the uncertainty, risks, and benefits associated with screening tests, environmental risk assessments, and drugs for treating chronic ailments. The public is left to sift through contradictory information to find the most "meaningful" health benefit and risk statistics presented to them by experts.

It's all a matter of "framing." We're all familiar with the importance of how you frame a question. In this case, the issue is how to frame the answers. Framing not only makes it possible to present the same risk results in different ways, it also leads physicians and patients to make different choices. They will tend to accept risks when information is presented positively (e.g., in terms of survival), but not when findings are presented negatively (e.g., in terms of mortality). Many patients will accept a drug when told there are no serious side effects for 98% of people. But if told that 2% of people do experience serious side effects, many of the same patients will refuse the drug. Same data, different framing, different decision.[2]

A 1999 study[3] analyzed physician-researcher decisions about whether or not to stop a hypothetical clinical trial. The decisions were influenced by how trial data were displayed and framed. As it turned out, not only does the presentation make a difference, but *it is more likely to bias in the direction of risk aversion.*[2]

Framing health benefit and risk data in a clear and concise format will reduce anxiety and controversy and encourage the public to be part of a sound, evidence-based decision-making process. Based on our analysis, it is not necessary to use intricate equations and numerical data to convey the meaning of health risks. Forthright verbal explanations can substitute for complex data tables and charts. Visual aids depicting recognizable situations can be very effective. Data can be framed in a manner that enables people to relate health statistics and risk analyses to familiar experiences.

A paradigm should be developed to portray health risks in an understandable and recognizable format. It should not be biased in the direction of risk aversion or risk acceptance. It should convey information about the differences in uncertainty between situations where cause and effect have been established and those where health decisions are based on risk factors and risk assessment.

When health benefits and risks are presented to the public, relative numbers and percentage comparisons should be avoided because of their distorting effect. Relative numbers can help governmental agencies and the medical community understand the national or international incidence of a disease. But relative numbers have virtually no value to individuals confronting critical health decisions. The focus should be on absolute benefits and risks, absolute risk reduction, and the number needed to treat, because these are the most important parameters for individual decisions.

Finally, people should be able to relate to the visual representation used to present uncertainty, risks, and benefits. An easily understood and consistent model should be developed so that health risks associated with different diseases or contaminants can be compared and evaluated in the context of each person's level of acceptable risk. We need to reframe the debate by providing informative, empowering materials that shatter the illusion of certainty.

Risk Characterization Theater

Since many individuals concerned with health risks have little or no medical or scientific background, the challenge is to develop a paradigm that effectively places health benefit and risk information in a familiar format that is easy to understand. In order for this model to be successful, it needs to include a visual display of data that enables the reader to understand and appreciate the outcome of health benefit and risk analyses and the uncertainty inherent in the reported results.

In other words, the reader should be able to look at an image and be able to see the risks and benefits from a screening test (e.g., mammography), a drug (e.g., Vioxx^{TM}), or a reduction in the level of an environmental contaminant (e.g., radon). The selected image should convey the absolute chance of benefit or injury, and be able to demonstrate at a glance that a 1 in 10 risk is very different from a 1 in 100,000 risk.

It occurred to us that a theater seating chart would be useful. Most of us are familiar with the crowd in a typical theater as a graphic illustration of a population grouping. With a seating capacity of 1,000, our hypothetical Risk Characterization Theater (RCT) makes it easy to illustrate a number of important values: the number of individuals who would benefit from screening tests, the number of individuals contracting a disease due to a specific cause (e.g., HIV and AIDS), and the merits of published risk factors (e.g., elevated cholesterol, exposure to low levels of environmental contaminants). If the necessary information is available, multiple RCTs can illustrate the uncertainty associated with the chance of a benefit or risk by showing a range of possible outcomes (examples are shown in Chap. 5). Ecological risks can also be portrayed using the same theater model.

We use our RCT to illustrate the specific case studies in this book, but we believe it is applicable to a larger set of situations involving health benefit and risk analyses. We use it to represent benefits and risks in a way that avoids bias and facilitates understanding. In each instance, absolute risk

(AR) and absolute risk reduction (ARR) will be calculated if the necessary data are available. Our primary motivation is to present health benefit and risk information to the public in an objective and useful format.

In every case study, the results we present come from research conducted by recognized experts in their field. Since many of these issues are controversial and contentious, we understand that there may be other experts who disagree with the data sets used to determine AR and ARR. Even so, using the RCT model will provide those who disagree with a framework to present alternatives to the public. This way, the people who are affected can participate in discussions and dialogue with the professionals who design risk-reducing treatments and interventions.

Mammograms and Breast Cancer

The Mammogram RCT (Fig. 3.1) illustrates the benefits of using mammograms as a screening test for breast cancer. A comprehensive analysis of Swedish women conducted by two Danish scientists (see discussion in Chap. 2), found that women who have had biennial mammograms have an

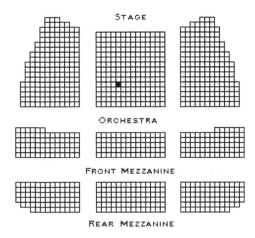

Fig. 3.1. The single darkened seat in the Mammogram RCT represents the 1 woman out of 1,000 who is likely to benefit from mammogram screening (as per the results of the Danish study discussed in Chap. 2) when compared to 1,000 women who did not have mammograms

Absolute Risk Reduction (ARR) of 0.1% or 1/1,000 when compared to women who did not have mammograms.

Our Mammogram RCT is filled with 1,000 women who have had biennial mammograms. The darkened seat represents the one woman out of 1,000 who would benefit from early cancer detection during mammogram screening. The remaining 999 women (99.9%) would not benefit.

Looking at the Mammogram RCT helps us to imagine the level of benefits from mammography. Considering this level of benefit (1 in 1,000), we might suspect that different women could make different decisions about how appropriate this screening test is for them. Each woman's personal decision would be based on her own definition of acceptable risk.

HIV and AIDS

For comparison, let's use the RCT to illustrate a case where cause and effect have been established for a serious health problem.

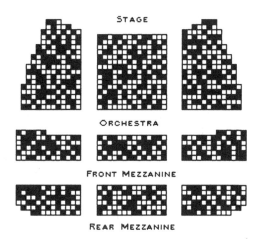

Fig. 3.2. The 500 darkened seats in the AIDS RCT represent the 500 out of 1,000 individuals who are likely to develop full-blown AIDS within ten years of becoming HIV-positive

Scientists have estimated that approximately 50% of individuals develop AIDS within 10 years after being infected with the HIV virus. The 1,000-seat AIDS RCT (Fig. 3.2) is filled with individuals infected with HIV. The darkened seats represent the number of them who would come down with AIDS within 10 years of infection. HIV has been demonstrated to be the cause of AIDS; therefore, HIV is always present when AIDS is diagnosed.

It is evident from the AIDS RCT that there is a strong correlation between being infected with HIV and the onset of AIDS. In this case the uncertainty is low and the predictability is high.

Many of the following chapters will include RCTs to illustrate the benefits and risks associated with selected screening tests, drugs, and exposure to environmental contaminants.

4. Assessing Human Health Risks from Environmental Contaminants

We have to expose the assumptions that go into risk assessments. We have to admit our uncertainties and confront the public with the complex nature of decisions about risk.

William D. Ruckelshaus[1]

The events and risk assessment results discussed and presented in this chapter are accurate in terms of location, organizations involved, analysis of data, and interpretation of results. The authors invented the reporter and EPA official as a more engrossing way to present this information.

There were over 1,500 irate and concerned people packed into a Northern California high school auditorium for a public hearing that would last for two and a half days. The purpose of the meeting was to discuss a recently released report which described the potential adverse health effects resulting from exposure to air emissions generated by two local pulp mills. The odors emanating from the pulp mills were certainly objectionable, but the primary reason all of these folks attended this hearing was to hear what the "experts" had to say about the possible increase in cancer or other diseases. In the weeks leading up to the hearing, not a day went by without an article on the front page of the local newspapers discussing not only health risks to local residents but also the economic implications for the region if the mills were forced to close. This was a classic confrontation of jobs versus health and the overlying concern of maintaining a quality environment.

The issues were not unique to this small California town, so what happened here would be of considerable interest to people throughout the country. That's why the editor-in-chief of a major San Francisco newspaper decided to do a series of articles highlighting concerns and impacts for different constituencies. The newspaper sent its chief environmental reporter, Joe Phelps, to cover the hearing and get background information from groups and individuals with different perspectives. This was the 1980s, a time when environmental risk assessment was a fledgling science and corporations were just starting to be held accountable for exceeding pollution standards. The stakes were high for all involved. Although there were marked differences in philosophy, goals, and objectives, it was generally assumed that science would drive the decision-making process.

Phelps had covered dozens of stories involving potential destruction of natural resources and impacts on human health. He understood the need to be objective and to avoid allowing his paper's political perspective to slant the way scientific results were presented. This required a rather sophisticated understanding of the scientific issues being debated and the ability to communicate complex issues to the general public – skills not all journalists possessed. He also understood that his employer was in the business of selling newspapers. This generally meant that the more dramatic and earthshaking the news, the better. Even if he could convince his editor that anything but a balanced and objective treatment of an issue would be inappropriate, the article's headline would most likely lean to hyperbole and exaggeration because reporters often don't get to choose their own headlines.

Estimating Human Health and Environmental Risks

Before departing for the hearing, Phelps wanted assurance from his boss that he would have a high degree of control over the content of the articles and the wording of the headlines. He also asked for approval to research the history of environmental risk assessment, the specific contaminants emanating from the pulp mills, and the legitimacy of different and opposing perspectives. He was given the go-ahead, even though this would result in significant costs to the newspaper. The editor had been around long enough to know that there would be a lot of public interest in the issues, and that it would be worth it to cover the story thoroughly.

As he began digging into the subject, Phelps found that risk analysis and risk assessment have been around for a long time, but their application to environmental health is relatively recent. Historians believe the first professional risk assessors were from ancient Babylon (3200 B.C.) and functioned as consultants offering advice on risky, uncertain, or difficult decisions in life. Risk assessment has long been practiced in the insurance and banking worlds. However, applications to human health and safety only began to emerge in the 20th century. Risk analysis is now being used to evaluate and manage potential problems on a wide range of issues including natural resource damages and environmental hazards.

When Phelps arrived for the hearing, it became abundantly clear that the stakeholders' positions spanned the entire spectrum. Those concerned about their jobs didn't think the health risks were real, while those who came to the area for the environmental amenities had diametrically opposed views. Industry consultants concluded that the risk assessment confirmed the absence of an imminent, long-term, or substantial danger from the pulp mill emissions, while environmentalists and non-governmental organizations sided with the residents who valued the region's unique natural attributes. Federal, state, and local agencies appeared to be non-committal and straddling the fence. Phelps wondered how these opinions could be contradictory when each party was claiming the use of "sound science" to support its own interpretation. Then Phelps remembered something he had read in a textbook on environmental science, something that made such a strong impression that he never forgot it: *if risk assessment is the basis for characterizing human health risks, it would be prudent to assume that a high degree of uncertainty is associated with the research results and findings.*

Because the EPA and most other public and private groups conducting risk assessments use a "conservative" approach that tends to overestimate risks, human health risk assessments seldom approach the level of reliability normally expected of scientific findings. Indeed, many estimates are little more than educated guesses.[2,3] The resulting high level of uncertainty is in part due to the application of the "precautionary principle" or so-called Wingspread Declaration: "When an activity raises threats of harm to human health or the environment, precautionary measures should be taken even if some cause and effect relationships are not established scientifically."[4]

The intent of relying on this principle is to help protect human health, but history clearly shows that "precautionary measures" can also be blamed for significant harm and wasted resources. They have been responsible, in part, for a characterization of risks that is often confusing and misleading. The resulting risk assessment process has been criticized repeatedly for its inability to portray risks accurately from chronic exposures to low levels of contaminants. Risk estimates submitted in the Food and Drug Administration (FDA) proceedings on saccharin varied by more than a million fold.[5] Latin[6] indicated predictions of the hazards posed by TCE, a drinking water contaminant, varied by many millions. This range of variation is the same as not knowing whether one has enough money to buy a cup of coffee or pay off the national debt.[6]

Pulp mill operations have been associated with air, soil, surface water, and ground water contamination and very unpleasant odors. These odors are classified as a "nuisance" (undoubtedly more than that to those living or working near the mills), but other potential impacts to human health and the environment are considered to be far more serious. The hearing Phelps would cover was focused exclusively on air emissions and the potential for increased levels of cancer in the exposed population.

In order to determine cancer risks to the affected population in Northern California from the local pulp mills, data from the US Bureau of Census (1980) were used to estimate the current population in the defined study area. Then, county growth factors were used to estimate how many people would be present in the year 2060. Rather than assume a gradual increase in the population, it was conservatively assumed that the year 2060 population was present at the time of the analysis and that this population would be exposed for a lifetime of 70 years. The affected areas were carefully mapped on a grid, and population estimates within that grid were used to calculate the potential incidence of cancer.

Studies concluded that a hypothetical individual's maximum lifetime risk of contracting cancer from a 70-year inhalation exposure to pulp mill emissions would be 2 in 1,000,000. In other words, if 1,000,000 people were exposed to these emissions for 70 years, 2 additional people would theoretically contract cancer. Phelps noted that this risk estimate was considered "health protective." To illustrate this additional lifetime risk with the RCT concept, there would be 999 theaters (1,000 seats each) with no darkened seats and one theater with 2 darkened seats, as shown in Fig. 4.1.

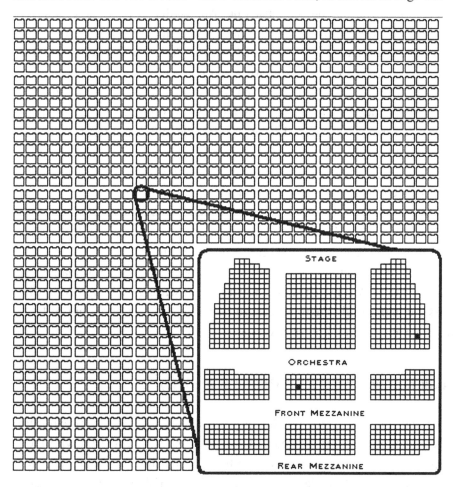

Fig. 4.1. The two darkened seats in a total of one thousand RCTs represent the 2 in a million additional cancers from lifetime exposure to emissions from the pulp mills in the California study

The presentation of the risk estimate differed depending on the particular risk analysis approach. The local newspapers and the environmental community were saying that the calculated risk of 2/1,000,000 individuals exceeded the California acceptable cancer risk standard of 1/1,000,000 by 100% – the relative risk difference, based on a comparison of the fractions' numerators 1 and 2. Using the same data, but a different approach, industry representatives concluded that the absolute risk would be 0.0002%. Using another statistical technique, industry determined that there would be approximately one cancer case in the area of concern if the population were exposed continuously for about 2,500 years. Phelps now understood that the manner in which this information was communicated made all the difference in the world. He realized that in order to get his arms around this issue, he needed to understand how the EPA, California, and other states developed their acceptable risk level – 1/1,000,000 – and what went into an environmental risk assessment. During his research he always kept in the back of his mind the caveat regarding the level of confidence associated with environmental risk assessments.

For a balanced view of the benefits and disadvantages of the risk assessment process, Phelps sought out J.W., an EPA expert from Region IX, which includes California. J.W. had a reputation for being a good scientist who was direct and upfront regarding controversial issues. Fortunately for Phelps, the EPA scientist was in town for the hearing. J.W. agreed to discuss the paper mill situation because he thought it was important to have accurate and unbiased press coverage.

Risk Management as a Political Activity

First and foremost, since this hearing was addressing risks from exposure to carcinogens, Phelps wanted to know how the EPA came up with their acceptable risk level of one in a million. Acceptable to whom? Was the designation of acceptable risk part of the formal risk assessment process? J.W. explained that there is no such thing as zero risk. Exposure to a few molecules would result in some risk value, albeit too low to be meaningful. Therefore, when the EPA began calculating and quantifying risks resulting from exposure to low levels of suspected carcinogens, it had to come up with a politically palatable – though arbitrary – number of cancers in the entire population that would be deemed acceptable.

The EPA concluded that acceptable would range from 1 in ten thousand to 1 in a million over a 70-year lifetime. J.W. stressed that establishing an allowable excess risk level is a value judgment. It is not based on scientific analysis. The acceptable risk spanned a very large range. Predictably, industry backed the more lenient value of 1 in 10,000, while the environmental community supported the more conservative value of 1 in 1,000,000. In the end, the EPA gave the states the authority to select their own acceptable risk value within the EPA's range, and most chose the 1 in 1,000,000 level. This means that from the perspective of health protection, practicality, and cost effectiveness, an additional 300 cancers across the country over a lifetime are acceptable, considering that the US population is about 300 million.

This led Phelps to ask about the acceptable risk level and its relationship to the formal risk assessment process. J.W. answered that the designation of acceptable risks fell into the category of risk management, a process related to, but not part of, a scientific risk assessment. "Many people who should know better," said J.W., "think that acceptable risks are scientifically derived."

In the context of human health risk assessments, risk management involves weighing policy alternatives and selecting the most appropriate regulatory actions or medical interventions to reduce the risk. He defined it this way: *risk management is a political activity that balances interests and values to determine whether human health risks should be considered unacceptable or tolerable.*

The primary objective of risk management is to integrate the analytical results of risk assessment with social, economic, and political concerns as illustrated in Fig. 4.2. The left circle represents the components of risk assessment that evaluate a risk in terms of the nature and consequences of the adverse impact, the potential causes of the adverse impact, and the likelihood that the adverse impact will occur. The knowledge from risk assessment is used in risk management (illustrated by the right circle in Fig. 4.2) to select the appropriate regulatory action. This sharp distinction between the scientific process of risk assessment and the social policy dimensions of risk management is reflected in the EPA's guidelines, which state that risk assessments must "use the most scientifically appropriate interpretation" and should "be carried out independently from considerations of the consequences of regulatory action."[7]

Phelps then asked about the values derived from scientific risk assessments and how they compared to the acceptable risk values. In the case of the pulp mills, J.W. explained, scientists concluded that the cancer risk from lifetime exposure to airborne pulp mill emissions was 2/1,000,000, clearly greater than 1/1,000,000. How was this value obtained? How sure were the scientists of their results? Impressed by the questions, J.W. thought a little background information would be helpful.

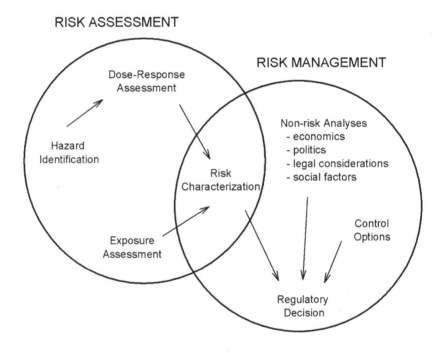

Fig. 4.2. Comparison of risk assessment and risk management

Risk Assessment as a Scientific Process

The use of risk assessment to characterize adverse effects on human health has become a well-accepted and widely-used approach by environmental regulatory agencies and the medical community. It is generally defined this way: *human health risk assessment is a scientific process that evaluates, derives, and predicts the probability of an adverse effect of an agent (chemical, physical, or biological), industrial process, technology, or biological condition (cholesterol level, blood pressure, obesity) on individuals and populations.*

For some contaminants and exposure conditions, it has been easy to predict acute and chronic health risks. This is true when historical statistical data are available and when the causal connection between injury and exposure to the contaminant is easy to demonstrate. For example, hundreds of people have died as a result of eating fish from mercury-contaminated coastal areas in Japan.[8] Adverse health effects from lead exposure are well-documented. After ingesting rice oil contaminated with polychlorinated biphenyls (PCBs), many individuals in Japan reported health effects that included severe dermatitis, excessive pigmentation of the skin, aches and pain, peripheral nerve damage, and severe headaches.[9] In all these cases, the link between contaminant exposure and effect was strong, either because the situation involved acute toxicity and the adverse effect was realized shortly after exposure, or because chronic effects were clearly related to increased dose and specific exposure pathways, such as inhalation, ingestion, or contact with skin.

Predicting health risks from exposure to environmental carcinogens is more problematic. In terms of potential cancers resulting from exposure to air emissions from the pulp mills in California, the contaminants of primary concern were determined to be chloroform, benzene, and dioxin. There was ample evidence to list each as a carcinogen. Phelps wanted to know how that evidence was gathered, analyzed, evaluated, and interpreted. J.W. thought that was a fair question, but he warned that he only had time to explain the basic principles of risk assessment. After all, there were entire books devoted to each step in the risk assessment process.

Steps in Risk Assessment

The standard paradigm for environmental human health risk assessment consists of four steps, as shown in Fig. 4.2.[10] This model is used, in one form or another, by practically all institutions conducting risk assessments in the US.

The four steps are:

1. Hazard Identification: does the contaminant cause an undesirable effect?
2. Dose-Response Assessment: what is the relationship between the contaminant dose and the adverse health effect?
3. Exposure Assessment: what exposures are experienced or anticipated under different conditions?
4. Risk Characterization: what is the estimated occurrence of the adverse effect in a population?

The first step in the risk assessment process, *hazard identification*, involves evaluating data on the kinds of health effects that occur after exposure to an environmental insult. The purpose is to determine whether it is scientifically correct to infer that toxic effects observed in one setting will also occur in other settings. For example, are substances found to be carcinogenic in experimental animals likely to have the same effect in humans?

Chemical toxic properties are usually determined through controlled laboratory studies with various animal species and through studies of people who happen to have been exposed to a chemical (epidemiological investigations). If all the data point clearly in a single direction, decisions about the nature of toxicity are easy. Often, however, there are conflicting and ambiguous findings. When this happens, scientists cannot be certain about environmental risks. Nevertheless, the present focus of environmental regulations is to protect humans from exposure to trace levels of potentially hazardous contaminants over long time periods, *even when adverse effects are not evident.*

The most common and straightforward way to measure acute toxic effects is by determining a single oral dose that will kill half of the test organisms within 24 hours. This dose, the lethal dose at which 50% of the exposed population will die, is known as LD_{50}. Chemicals requiring a higher concentration to achieve the same lethal effect are less toxic.

At this point, Phelps asked how an LD_{50} would be determined when exposure was by inhalation – the situation that would be discussed at the public hearing. J.W. explained that the lethal concentration of a suspected contaminant in the air that will cause the death of 50% of the exposed population is called an LC_{50}, and is a measure of acute toxicity for gases. It generally allows for a time of inhalation of about four hours.

Studies of hazard identification also attempt to answer the question, "does the agent cause cancer in test animals?" In these studies, animals are exposed to relatively high doses of the test chemical and observed to see if tumors develop. This is because the chance of a test animal getting cancer at the lower concentrations found in the environment is extremely small, so low-dose tests are not likely to yield positive results for observing a health hazard.

After developing an understanding of the toxicity exhibited by substances of concern in the hazard identification step, the next step is to estimate the *dose-response relationship*. This determines the relation between the dose of a contaminant received and the incidence of an adverse health effect. This step estimates the likelihood that a person will be adversely impacted by a given dose of a contaminant, and it relies primarily on data obtained from animal studies. With dose-response information, researchers are able to compare scientifically calculated health risks with acceptable levels of exposure.

After carrying out animal studies to calculate an LD_{50} or an LC_{50}, scientists expose test organisms to smaller and smaller doses and for longer periods of time in an attempt to establish a dose-response relationship. For non-carcinogens, it is assumed that there is a threshold below which there is no adverse effect. This is called the *no observable adverse effect level* (NOAEL). J.W. showed Phelps a chart to illustrate the possible behavior for a non-carcinogenic substance in an animal study (Fig. 4.3). Curve A illustrates a simple dose-response relationship for a theoretical non-carcinogenic substance. As the dose decreases, the response also decreases until it reaches a point where a response cannot be measured or observed: this is the "threshold," or NOAEL. Exposure to non-carcinogenic contaminants is generally evaluated in terms of a *reference dose* (RfD). An RfD is an estimate of a daily exposure that is assumed to be without adverse effect after a lifetime of exposure. RfDs are established from all available toxicological data for hundreds of chemicals.

RfDs are calculated by dividing NOAELs by:

1. Uncertainty factors – quality and type of animal study used to calculate NOAELs
2. Modifying factors – depend on the quality of the toxicological database for a particular chemical; these factors can range from 10 to 10,000

Phelps assumed the selection of uncertainty factors and modifying factors was not exact. He was right on target. By this time, Phelps already had pages of notes about the steps in assessing health risks. Yet his friend from the EPA continued. For carcinogens, it is assumed that there is no such threshold; even a single molecule can trigger a reaction, such as the alteration of DNA, which can lead to cancer.

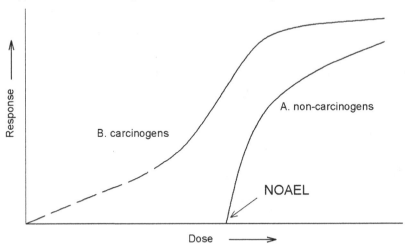

Hypothetical Dose-Response Curves for Carcinogens and Non-carcinogens

Fig. 4.3. *Curve A* represents a dose-response curve for non-carcinogens. It assumes a threshold level where no observable adverse effect occurs (*NOAEL*). *Curve B* represents a dose-response curve for carcinogens. It assumes no threshold. The dashed line is the area that is extrapolated and determined using models

Observation of chronic effects, like cancer, can only be determined with long-term studies. The researchers must first find a dose in test animals that won't result in an acute response like death. Since environmental levels of contaminants are generally very low, experimental animals exposed to environmental levels don't usually develop cancer. So tests must be conducted at artificially elevated exposure levels that are high enough to have an effect, yet low enough to be non-lethal over the lifetime of the test animal. Researchers then use models to extrapolate the high-dose test results to environmentally relevant concentrations. The curve labeled "B" in Fig. 4.3 illustrates a dose-response curve for a theoretical carcinogen. The dashed area on the curve indicates the low dose range where there were no data from animal experiments. This portion of the line was generated by model predictions. Phelps asked if the use of specific models was generally accepted by experts in this field. J.W. smiled. Analyzing risks associated with chronic exposures and toxicity is a complicated and multifaceted task. Three major extrapolations are involved: animal to human, high dose to low dose, and normal-risk to high-risk segment of the population.[4,11] "The truth is," J.W. added, "none of these mathematical models are chemical-specific." Instead, each is just based on general theories of carcinogenesis. Scientifically derived data cannot, with any degree of certainty, prove or disprove any of the models.

Phelps learned that benzene, chloroform, and dioxin had been characterized as human carcinogens based on evidence from epidemiological and animal studies. He also learned that if a pollutant is a carcinogen that also causes other health effects, regulations are generally calculated for cancer, since that will result in a more restrictive level of acceptable exposure. The idea is that if you protect against cancer, you automatically protect against other health endpoints.

Once the dose-response relationship is determined for the carcinogens of concern at the pulp mills, the third risk assessment step must be taken: *exposure assessment*. This involves determining the number of people exposed and the magnitude and duration of the exposure to a contaminant present in the environment. Exposure assessment is also used to estimate hypothetical exposures that might arise from new releases of a contaminant or releases of new chemicals into the environment. Establishing the important routes of exposure, such as through ingestion of food and water, breathing of air, and contact with skin, is another component of exposure assessment. Finally, the exposure assessment often includes data on the size, nature, and classes of human populations exposed.

Estimation of contaminant concentrations in environmental media is a necessary step to determine the dose received by the exposed population. Since measurements of the transport and ultimate fate of contaminants can be difficult, time-consuming, and costly, it is common to rely on mathematical models to predict contaminant behavior and obtain exposure information. Knowledge of the chemical movement and behavior obtained during exposure assessment can often be used to identify feasible control options for eliminating or limiting exposure. Examples include capping to contain a contaminant, or a biological or chemical treatment system to degrade the chemical.

After the information from the first three risk assessment steps is evaluated, it is then communicated to all concerned during the fourth and final step, *risk characterization*. This is the process of combining the dose-response and exposure assessments to estimate the incidence of a health effect under the various conditions of human exposure to a contaminant. For a carcinogen, the risk estimate is expressed as the likelihood of additional lifetime cancers (e.g., 1/1,000,000). For non-carcinogens, risk is described by a hazard quotient (HQ) that is the ratio of the contaminant dose over a specified time period to the RfD derived for a similar exposure period.

Of all the four steps in the formal, scientific risk assessment process, the one that consistently gets short shrift is risk characterization. That is unfortunate, because some would say that risk characterization is by far the most important of all. Risk managers, including government agencies and politicians, universally rely on characterized risk values to decide whether funds should be allocated to combat unacceptable human health problems and whether restrictions should be placed on industrial sources.

Risk Communication

For the potentially carcinogenic air emissions associated with the California pulp mills, risk is estimated and steps are taken to manage this level of characterized risk. The decision could have serious consequences for residents, including pulp mill workers. Groups that conduct environmental risk assessments or have a vested interest in the outcome – industry, labor, the environmental community – are often well-funded and politically connected. They are all too ready to praise assessment results that serve their interests or wage war against results that don't align with their agendas, retaining consultants and challenging findings by promoting alternate models or methods.

The many steps of the risk assessment process can justify a wide range of "scientifically sound" decisions and approaches. The risk can be characterized as anything from trivial to dire. J.W. demonstrated with a number of possible pronouncements:

- An additional 2 out of 1,000,000 individuals will die from a lifetime exposure to benzene, chloroform and dioxin emissions from the two California pulp mills.
- If the entire US population were exposed over their lifetime to emissions like those from the two California pulp mills, there would be approximately 600 additional cancer victims.
- Benzene, chloroform, and dioxin are carcinogenic in rats and mice, and it is prudent public health policy to assume they are also carcinogenic in humans.
- Benzene, chloroform, and dioxin are carcinogenic in rats and mice. The application of low-dose extrapolation models and human exposure estimates suggest that the range of lifetime risks in humans is zero to 2 deaths per 1,000,000 persons exposed; therefore, the percent death rate ranges from 0% to 0.0002%.
- The increase in cancer cases in individuals living near the two California pulp mills will range from one cancer case every 2,333 years to one case every 3,500 years. There is an equal probability that there will be zero cases of cancer from exposure to these pulp mill emissions.

"All of these statements are 'scientifically accurate,'" J.W. said. "All ignore, to one degree or another, the caveat to include and discuss the uncertainty in the characterization of health risks. Risk managers, politicians, newspaper reporters like you, environmental organizations, and industry trade associations can and most likely will 'spin' risk values to suit their different agendas."

As it turned out, there were no surprises at the hearing. As J.W. predicted, each presentation touted that particular stakeholder's version of the truth. All claimed to be based on sound scientific evidence. None discussed the level of certainty and confidence in the findings.

After mulling over the situation, Phelps realized he had found a focus for his article. It wouldn't have any shock value – and therefore probably wouldn't sell any extra newspapers – but someone needed to explain how human health risks are assessed and how the manner in which risks are characterized can lead to a wide range of possible outcomes.

The next chapter will provide more detail on the limitations and uncertainty associated with characterizing human health benefits and risks. Until we find a way to incorporate and interpret uncertainty in the final characterization of health benefits and risks, scientific information will not drive the decision-making process. It may look as if it does, but that will most certainly be a fantasy.

5. The Sources of Uncertainty

Increasingly we must rely on experts when we make decisions. It is often hard to be sure we understand exactly what they are telling us. It is harder still to know what to do when different experts appear to be telling us different things. If we insist they tell us about the uncertainty of their judgments, we will be clearer about how much they think they know and whether they really disagree.

M. Granger Morgan and Max Henrion[1]

A health benefit is defined as the chance of improvement or positive outcome from a medical screening test or drug intervention. A health risk is the chance of harm from a medical treatment program or exposure to an environmental contaminant. All health benefits and risks involve chance or probability, because we can never know the future with complete certainty.[2,3]

Previous chapters have discussed how the estimates of the probability of a benefit or adverse outcome are made with more or less confidence. When there is a clear cause and effect relationship, such as in the case of HIV and AIDS, the confidence level is high. When a cause and effect relationship has not been identified, there is a lower level of confidence in predictions about the possible benefits or adverse effects to human health.

In spite of this variable confidence factor, the possibility of a health benefit or risk is usually presented as a single numerical value. We can't tell if that single value is the worst-case scenario, the sunniest situation, or a number that gives a more realistic estimate of the benefit or risk. Nor can we tell how reliable that single value is. Is it "virtually sure" or merely a "best guess?"

In short, reporting a benefit or risk value as a single number often creates an illusion of certainty. This chapter discusses the many sources of uncertainty in characterizing health benefits and risks.

Why is Uncertainty Left Out?

One reason reports about health benefits and risks don't mention uncertainty is because it leads to anxiety. We look to our experts for concrete answers, especially about our health. So to avoid making us uncomfortable, doctors and scientists give us the simplified answers we want to hear.

The need on the part of authorities to project power and control is a second major reason uncertainty is not acknowledged. Federal and state environmental regulatory agencies are responsible for protecting the public from exposure to environmental contaminants. People want to know in absolute terms what contaminant levels are safe and what levels are harmful. So the regulatory agencies are under pressure to establish clear-cut environmental cleanup goals. However, experts can't exactly pinpoint "the safe level," because there is too much uncertainty in the analysis. Instead, they can only try to narrow down the range of their answer. Rather than risk sounding "wishy-washy" while trying to explain how any one of an entire range of "safe levels" has an equal chance of being protective, it's easier for regulatory agencies to deal in single-number cleanup goals. And it's also easiest if these single-number goals apply to the entire universe of environmental contamination situations, however unrealistic that may be.

How does Understanding Uncertainty Help Us?

Why bother delving into the complex subject of uncertainty? There are several good reasons to make the effort.[1]

First, the level of uncertainty gives us an indication of what we know and what we don't know. Public health experts conduct epidemiological studies to quantify impacts on human health using established principles of their profession. Medical experts conduct clinical trials using scientific principles to establish the efficacy of a screening test or new drug. The uncertainty helps identify which portions of a study need additional attention. Science uses uncertainty to design better experiments to probe the unknown.

Second, an explanation of the uncertainty of a study's results helps the public to understand the health benefit and risk numbers that are generated and the level of confidence in them. This enables us to make better-informed decisions.

Third, uncertainties encountered in previous health studies help tell us how much confidence to put in future studies. For example, the measured behavior of past releases of contaminants in our water and soil can be used to evaluate how new chemical releases are likely to behave. Similarly, the outcome of a clinical trial to establish the efficacy of a new drug with one subgroup of the population can be used to prescribe treatment for members of the entire population. In cases like these, it's essential to understand how confident researchers were of the results obtained in those previous studies.

Fourth, quantifying the uncertainty helps reveal the limits of our knowledge and its usefulness in making decisions. A single benefit or risk number can lead to misguided societal and individual decision-making, while knowing the whole range of possible outcomes helps us frame our options. For example, consistent agreement among different studies and an established cause and effect relationship would point to a neater decision, or at least clear advice. But when the outcomes involve risk factors and if there is controversy among the studies, the uncertainty is high and the proper course of action is less clear. Will your decision be based on "scientists are almost positive that..." or on "doctors think that maybe..." or on something in between? Would you make the same choice in every case? Unless you know something quantitative about uncertainty, you can't even tell what category you're in.

Key Uncertainties in Risk Assessment

As discussed in the previous chapter, conclusions about human health risks come from a multi-step risk assessment process:

- hazard identification,
- dose-response assessment,
- exposure assessment,
- and risk characterization

Uncertainty can occur at all levels of the analysis,[4] and it is carried through to the final risk calculation.

Even though EPA risk assessment guidelines are written to make this uncertainty clear, the details of it are almost always lost. As a result, the illusion of certainty has become firmly entrenched in the process of environmental and medical risk characterization. The following sections highlight the key uncertainties in each step of the risk assessment process. Although the discussion focuses on environmental contamination, similar kinds of uncertainties occur in epidemiological studies and in clinical trials characterizing the benefits of a new drugs or diagnostic tests.

Uncertainties in Hazard Identification

Some of the generally recognized kinds of uncertainty in the hazard identification phase of human health risk assessments are listed in Box 5.1. A few areas deserve to be discussed in more detail.

Animal studies are often used to determine if a chemical is likely to be toxic in humans, based on the assumption that effects seen in animals can be expected to occur in humans as well. This makes sense when humans and test animals show similarities in physiology, anatomy, and biochemistry. But there are a number of exceptions that make animal toxicity studies problematic, so great care must be taken when inferring human toxicity from animal toxicological study results.

Box 5.1. Generally recognized sources of uncertainty in hazard identification
- Extrapolating data from animal experiments to humans
- Interpreting the relevance of tumors that appear in control animals (animals not exposed to dose of a chemical)
- Attempting to determine if benign tumors will eventually become carcinogenic
- Extrapolating normal risk to a high-risk segment of the population (children, the elderly)
- Determining if the selected test animals metabolize chemicals the same way as humans do
- Determining if there is a high level of statistical significance in the increase of tumor incidence in treated vs. control animals
- Making sure an appropriate number of dose levels was used to develop a well-characterized dose-response relationship
- Ensuring that control animals are of the same species, strain, sex, age, and state of health as the treated animals
- Ensuring that the route of exposure resembles that through which humans will be exposed
- Determining what level of dose should be given over a lifetime when assessing carcinogenicity
- Making sure that there is a sufficient understanding of the mechanisms of carcinogenicity so that the selected doses provide meaningful results
- Ensuring that all aspects of the conduct and interpretation of toxicity tests are handled properly (e.g., adequate experimental design, careful observation of animals, dose of test compound correctly determined by chemical analysis, adequate statistical tests)

There are many reasons why a chemical may cause certain kinds of toxic effects in animals but not humans. One is the fact that very high doses are often administered to test animals, while much lower doses are encountered in the real world by humans. Also, high doses administered during animal testing can lead to chronic tissue damage that will not occur at low doses.[5] Consequently, animal studies with high doses can easily overestimate the risk at normal levels. Differences in the severity or type of toxic effects between animals and humans also result from differences in eating characteristics, affected tissues, digestion rates, ability to repair DNA, and the amount of time the chemical is present in the organism.

Epidemiological studies are also used to identify hazards. An epidemiological approach examines the relationship between exposure and health effects in actual human populations. Such studies have the advantage of involving human populations that experience exposure at normal environmental levels and represent a range of variability in susceptibility and behavior. But it can be difficult to link an observed effect to a specific cause. It can even be difficult to determine if there is an effect at all. Another challenge is estimating the actual dose received by the individuals being monitored, because there are many exposure pathways, and environmental concentrations can vary over time. What's more, humans are typically exposed to a number of different chemicals, and our knowledge of compound interactions is poor. All these factors are sources of uncertainty in epidemiological studies.

Another source of uncertainty in epidemiological studies is that very large sample sizes are generally required in order to detect a small increase in risk compared with the control group. This is best illustrated using a hypothetical example.

An epidemiological study involves 5,000 people who drink water from a well that is found to contain low levels of a carcinogenic contaminant. A control group of 5,000 people is identified. They obtain their drinking water from a different well that does not contain the contaminant. These two populations are surveyed for ten years. Of the 5,000 people drinking water with the contaminant, 4,990 people remain cancer-free after ten years. The number of healthy individuals in the group of 5,000 people who drink water without the contaminant is found to be 4,991. In short, ten people from the group drinking water with the contaminant develop cancer and nine people drinking from the other well are afflicted by cancer. The difference between the two groups is one additional cancer occurrence. It would be one thing if 100 people drinking contaminated water got cancer, compared to 9, but in this situation it is difficult to prove with much certainty that the one additional cancer was caused by the contaminant. Because the changes are small relative to the large number of people in the study (one additional cancer out of 5,000 people), repeating the study is likely to yield a different outcome. Another study might find that the number of healthy persons is the same for the two groups, or instead that the difference between the two groups is three additional cancer occurrences. The key point is there is little confidence in any of these results – zero, or one, or three additional cancers – due to the intrinsic uncertainty in these types of studies. To make matters worse, it takes a considerable amount of money and effort to conduct an epidemiological study, making it difficult to repeat it for the sake of improving the level of certainty and confidence in the results.

Uncertainties in Dose-Response Relationship

Since epidemiological studies do not usually provide reliable data to link doses and health effects, quantitative dose-response assessments usually rely on animal studies. But the EPA[6] and others[7,8] have long acknowledged that animal studies raise a number of serious problems that result in uncertainty:

1. Animals are usually exposed at high doses, and effects at environmentally relevant low doses must be predicted using models based on theories about the nature of the dose-response relationship;
2. Animals and humans often differ in response to an environmental insult due to differences in size and metabolism; and
3. The human population is heterogeneous, with some individuals likely to be more susceptible than others.

Mathematical dose-response models are sometimes used to assess human health risks. Though they have become more sophisticated in recent years, ambiguity and overall uncertainty remain disturbingly high. Model-generated estimates of responses correspond well to actual carcinogenic responses observed in animal experiments using high doses, but experimental animals exposed to environmental levels of carcinogens rarely develop cancer, making it impossible to assess the accuracy of the dose-response models at environmental levels. There may be more uncertainty in the models used in dose-response assessments than in any of the other steps in the risk assessment process.

Researchers are trying to determine exactly how compounds interact with our bodies to cause cancer. Carcinogenic effects can occur at very low levels of exposure, but since these mechanisms aren't yet clear, there is considerable uncertainty regarding the amount of a contaminant needed to convert a normal cell to a cancerous one. For example, scientists think that some carcinogens ("initiators") act during the initial stages of cancer and others ("promoters") are more influential during later stages. There are also physiological differences among subpopulations and individuals that determine susceptibility to risk. The EPA assumes that there is no "threshold" for carcinogens. To protect health, the Agency applies many safety factors to account for the uncertainties and thereby comes up with extremely conservative estimates of the acceptable exposure levels.

Uncertainties in Exposure Assessment

The mere existence of a chemical in the environment does not in itself represent a human health or ecological risk. For a risk to exist there must be not only a source of chemical release, but also a human or ecological receptor to get exposed and an environmental pathway connecting the source and receptor. If a risk is present, it may be reduced or eliminated by removing the source or receptor, or by interrupting the pathway.

There are many types of uncertainties that pertain to exposure assessment.[9] Components that contribute to uncertainty include the level of human exposure, the number and type of people likely to be exposed, and the possible exposure pathways.[10,11] The uncertainties that arise in quantifying the health effects in human receptors from exposure to contaminants have already been discussed. We'll now look at some of the uncertainties associated with contamination sources and with the chemicals' movement through and reactions in the environment.

Often, information about contaminant sources is incomplete. Locations are difficult to pinpoint, the history of contaminant releases is not documented, variations in mass or concentration distributions of contaminants are not clear, and the precise chemical composition of a released contaminant is unknown. Subsurface soil, rock, and water properties vary over space and time. Variability in the material properties gives rise to variability in the subsurface distribution of a contaminant. These uncertainties can be reduced by studying the site, reviewing past records, and monitoring long-term contaminant behavior, but some uncertainties are likely to remain.

Another cause of uncertainty is measurement error during sampling and analysis. It is not possible to gather complete knowledge about the soil or rock properties or about the nature of past chemical releases in the environment, so some uncertainty is always present in estimating chemical concentrations that exist in the subsurface.

In order to estimate contaminant concentrations that may reach human or ecological receptors over a period of time, scientists try to determine how contaminants move and react in the environment. To conduct this phase of risk assessment, they rely on measurements of chemical behavior in the environment and on predictions generated by using contaminant fate and transport models. This pathway characterization is fraught with uncertainty. First, there are many processes, such as water movement, transfer from water to air, dissolution of a solid into water, chemical precipitation and reaction, biodegradation, or binding to solids, that alter the movement and distribution of a contaminant. Second, the properties of the earth's crust are highly variable. This variability will alter how fast water and contaminants can move and react underground. Field measurements that are used to understand contaminant behavior are all subject to uncertainty because of sampling and analytical errors.

Development of quantitative fate and transport models requires an understanding of the physical, chemical, and biological processes that control the movement and reactions of contaminants along pathways. The models are representations of reality, and limitations in our understanding of the processes lead to uncertainty in the model structure and predictions. The models that estimate environmental exposure levels require many input parameters to describe the various geologic, hydraulic, chemical, and biological processes. These input parameters come from direct measurements or can be inferred by fitting mathematical models to field or laboratory measurements. Any uncertainty in the measurements is carried through to the model output.

The variability of the environment, uncertainties in the ability to define physical, chemical, and biological fate and transport processes, and limitations of fate and transport models make it difficult to know the precise distribution of a contaminant released from a source. This inevitably leads to uncertainty in estimating concentrations to which a receptor is exposed.

While the models continue to be refined and recalibrated as more field data are collected, the uncertainty in most aspects of pathway characterization remains high.

The case study involving two California pulp mills presented in Chap. 4 illustrates some of the uncertainties in exposure assessment. People were concerned about the potential for adverse health effects from exposure to the air emissions from the mills. But any judgment about risk would be clouded by uncertainties in all the factors listed in Box 5.2.

Box 5.2. Example sources of uncertainty in exposure assessment for the Chap. 4 case study involving two California pulp mills

- Data on production, quantities, and release of benzene, chloroform, and dioxin from these specific pulp mills.
- Knowledge of the movement, distribution, and fate of the released compounds in the atmosphere.
- The transport and fate of these air contaminants when they come in contact with soil, water, and sediments.
- Factors controlling the movement, persistence, and degradation of these carcinogens.
- Information on methods of human intake and human contact, including contact by sensitive populations such as children and the elderly.

Uncertainties in Ecological Risk Assessment

Most of the uncertainties that affect human health risk assessments also influence the determination of the possible impacts of human activities on the environment.[13] This exercise is called ecological risk assessment (ERA). The same uncertainties surrounding contaminant sources and pathways are present when determining the exposure levels for plants and animals. As in human health studies, the mobility of organisms and the variability of a contaminant in space and time produce considerable uncertainty about how much of the contaminant contacts the organism in the ecosystem. As with establishing human health impacts, there is considerable uncertainty in the results from toxicity tests to establish potential adverse effects on the wide variety of ecological receptors.

Two additional types of uncertainty are unique to ERA.[13] First, ERA must address a vast array of organisms, from many species of plants and fungi to crabs, starfish, worms, and of course vertebrates like fish, frogs, lizards, birds, and humans. The diversity of physiological processes and chemical sensitivities among these organisms is much greater than the differences between human beings. Second, it is hard to discern the effects of contaminants on the stability and long-term health of the ecosystem. The interplay among the different species and the response to contaminants on an ecosystem level are poorly understood. There are great uncertainties in the scale of disturbances that can be tolerated by ecosystems. Chapter 14 provides an expanded discussion with examples of the uncertainties surrounding ERA.

Approaches for Coping with Uncertainty in Risk Characterizations

The integration of several steps for risk assessment means that the uncertainties in each step are combined and compounded in health risk analysis. The overall uncertainty here is often much greater than in other physical sciences. As the risk gets smaller, the uncertainty sharply increases and the predictability of the exposure causing an adverse effect decreases. The impact of the uncertainty on predictability can be illustrated using the Risk Characterization Theater (RCT) graphic. Let's use the RCT to compare the uncertainty in the high risk AIDS example and the low risk pulp mills example.

In the case of HIV causing AIDS, the 500 darkened seats in the AIDS RCT shown in Fig. 5.1 show that approximately 50% of individuals develop AIDS within 10 years after being infected with the HIV virus. If the number of darkened seats increases or decreases by 10 to reflect uncertainty in the population affected, the chance of developing AIDS essentially remains the same at 1/2 (high predictability). The multiple RCTs in Fig. 5.1 show how uncertainty can be represented with the RCT graphic.

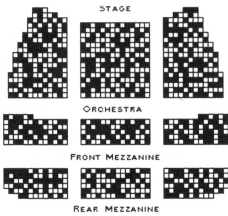

500 darkened seats - risk is 1/2

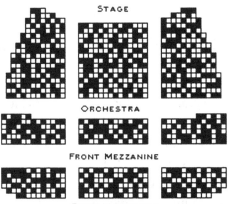

510 darkened seats - risk essentially 1/2

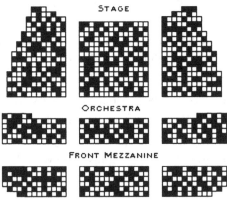

490 darkened seats - risk essentially 1/2

Now look at Fig. 5.2 for another example of visualizing uncertainty. These RCTs represent the case of exposure to pulp mill air emissions and the risk for additional lifetime cancers. Imagine the same uncertainty as in the HIV/AIDS example, a possible increase or decrease of 10 cancer cases, shown with darkened seats. But this time, the uncertainty results in more than a ten-fold range of estimated risk. Given the uncertainty in human health risk assessment, an increase or decrease of 10 cancers would not be unusual. Therefore, in this case there is an equal chance that the risk would approach zero, as reflected by the complete absence of darkened seats in Fig. 5.2c. The RCT graphics with 12 seats vs. 2 seats vs. 0 seats dramatize the fact that the estimated risk for the pulp mill example has much lower predictability.

Uncertainties in risk assessments are dealt with in one of three ways:[10]

1. using conservative cleanup goals (i.e., erring on the side of protecting health) in the case of environmental contamination,
2. conducting additional measurements and studies to refine under-standing and reduce uncertainty, or
3. performing a quantitative analysis of the uncertainty.

The first approach attempts to cope with uncertainty by using large safety factors and establishing ultra-conservative exposure levels or cleanup goals that are thought to provide sufficient protection of health or the ecosystem for a broad range of scenarios and conditions. These values are used to evaluate exposure situations rapidly so that those that clearly pose a negligible risk can be removed from the priorities list. If estimated risks from an exposure situation are unacceptable based on conservative assumptions, then more situation-specific data can be used to refine the analysis and develop a better characterization with less uncertainty. Though ultra-conservative screening levels are valuable for quickly dis-pensing with low-risk situations, they are often interpreted to be the only "safe" levels. This does not properly consider the conditions unique to

---

Fig. 5.1. (preceding page) An increase or decrease of 10 darkened seats to repre-sent uncertainty in the AIDS RCT (baseline shown in Fig. 3.2) doesn't appreciably alter the estimated risk for the presence of HIV causing AIDS

each situation and can lead to exaggeration of the risk and inefficient use of limited resources.

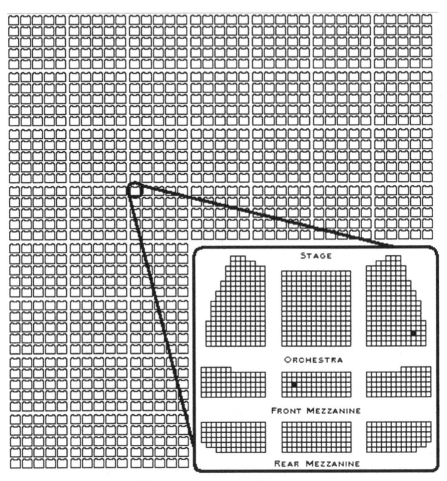

A. 2 darkened seats in 1,000 RCTs - risk is 2/1,000,000

Fig. 5.2. (this page and following pages) An increase (**B.**) or decrease (**C.**) of 10 darkened seats to represent uncertainty in the pulp mill air emissions RCT (baseline **A.** reproduced from Fig. 4.1) causes more than a 10 fold difference in the range of estimated risk for additional lifetime cancers

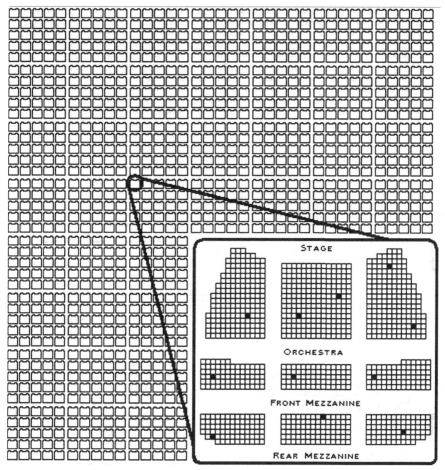

B. 12 darkened seats in 1,000 RCTs - risk is 12/1,000,000

The second approach for coping with uncertainty is to conduct additional measurements and studies to refine understanding and reduce uncertainty in risk estimates. Animal toxicity studies can be repeated to improve the confidence in identifying hazards, determining mechanisms of toxicity, and establishing dose-response relationships. Long-term monitoring can be used to provide data to define exposure pathways and contaminant concentrations better. Collecting additional data can help refine the assumptions on which the initial risk assessment was based, and further studies can put closer bounds on possible outcomes and establish more realistic risk values.

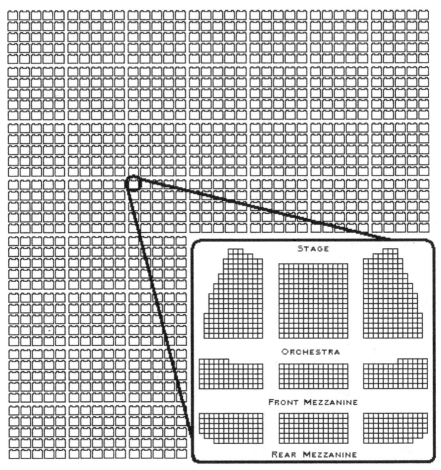

C. zero darkened seats in 1,000 RCTs - risk is less than 1/1,000,000

A third approach for coping with uncertainty is to conduct a quantitative analysis of the uncertainty itself. Almost all risk-based approaches have relied on the use of conservative assumptions and cleanup goals to account for uncertainty, yet they do not convey the degree of confidence or uncertainty in the risk estimate or provide information on how likely the risk may be. Formal uncertainty analysis of risk estimates can help to inform decision-makers as well as the general public about the level of conservatism actually contained in a risk assessment.

The technical details of formal uncertainty analysis can get complicated. The interested reader will find a short primer on statistical approaches to quantifying uncertainty in Appendix A. Several references are also available on this topic.[1,14,15]

A Persistent Illusion of Certainty

The risk assessment process must account for uncertainties regarding the contaminant sources, reactions in the environment, movement to potential receptors, and interactions with those receptors. These uncertainties can fuel disputes over the value of the risk estimate among regulatory agencies, polluters, and local communities. The toxicological and exposure assumptions, as well as the quality of the data used in the risk assessment, are often sources of considerable disagreement. Unfortunately, we usually only hear about the results of human health and environmental risk assessments, and not about the assumptions or the process.[16,17]

Determining the amount of uncertainty associated with a health benefit or risk number is not an easy task. In fact, it is a job for experts. And so these experts need to give sufficient descriptions of their rationale, procedures, data, and assumptions so that others – scientists, regulatory officials, and members of the public – can verify the information and better understand the work and results. Dr. George M. Gray, the current Director of the EPA Office of Research and Development, has recently articulated this goal.[18] Dr. Gray wants EPA scientists to provide formal, detailed explanations of uncertainty surrounding the health or environmental risk numbers they provide to policymakers, rather than offering a single number that is their best estimate.

The EPA and others familiar with limitations in the determination of human health risks always caution those interpreting risks to be sure the uncertainty is characterized fairly and accurately. Government documents, position papers, and textbooks often include caveats cautioning against the tendency to read too much into quantitative estimates. But in spite of all these admonitions, we usually characterize risk without ever discussing, explaining, or even acknowledging the related uncertainties. Reported final risk values then acquire an unmerited aura of definitive respectability. These values take on "a life of their own," and an illusion of certainty is created.

This chapter has focused on the uncertainties associated with health risks from environmental contamination. The epidemiological and clinical studies used to determine health benefits from medical screening tests and drugs generally have the same high level of uncertainty. In medical studies with humans, many things must be taken into account, such as age, smoking, alcohol consumption, and other lifestyle behaviors. In many instances, the outcomes of clinical trials in medicine may be no more certain than the extrapolations from animal studies for environmental contaminants.

In the medical and environmental case studies that follow, many of the RCTs have single values because we do not know the confidence limits on the numbers. The numbers are "ballpark values," and are the best we have. Where possible, we have acknowledged the uncertainty to help illustrate the application of the principles addressed in this chapter.

Part II

Case Studies

6. Vioxx™ and Heart Attacks

On the one hand, some patients and physicians will decide that any coxib-associated risk is too great when clear and safer alternatives exist.

D.H. Solomon and J. Avorn[1]

Issue

Vioxx™ (rofecoxib) was one of the drugs approved by the Food and Drug Administration for short-term treatment of acute pain and long-term treatment of rheumatoid arthritis and osteoarthritis. It seems, however, that these benefits came at a cost: higher risk of heart attack and stroke. A recent study estimated that Vioxx™ could have caused between 88,000 and 140,000 extra cases since its launch in 1999.[2] Another study suggested that millions of people may have been unnecessarily exposed to the risk of heart attacks by taking Vioxx™ and other medicines classified as non-steroidal anti-inflammatory drugs (NSAIDs).[3]

It appears that information on the benefits and risks of taking these drugs has not been clearly presented to the public. Problems with risk framing may be responsible for the less-than-helpful characterization of risks associated with these NSAIDs. Therefore, physicians, the FDA and other federal regulators, the media, and the public probably have an incomplete understanding of the risks and benefits.

The results of scientific studies provide good reason to assume there is an increased risk from cardiovascular events associated with taking Vioxx™. However, some patients seem unable to get relief with other drugs. Patients would, in all probability, benefit from an awareness of the specific risks and benefits associated with Vioxx™.

Background

In 1999, the drugs Vioxx™ and Celebrex™ were introduced. They soon became the most frequently prescribed new drugs in the US. By 2000, US sales exceeded 100 million prescriptions per year for $3 billion, and were still rising; sales of Celebrex™ alone reached $3.1 billion in 2001. These NSAIDs target an enzyme found to be responsible for inflammation and pain. This enzyme, COX-2 (cyclooxygenase 2 enzyme), is activated at sites of injury. It triggers the production of hormone-like substances called prostaglandins, which bring on painful inflammation. COX-2 inhibitors are drugs designed to block the activity of the COX-2 enzyme, thus relieving pain.[4]

Acceptance of Celebrex™ and Vioxx™ was rapid and widespread among physicians, largely due to the publication of two large trials: the Celecoxib Long-term Arthritis Safety Study (CLASS),[5] and the Vioxx™ Gastrointestinal Outcomes Research (VIGOR) study.[6] Both studies concluded that Celebrex™ and Vioxx™ were associated with significantly fewer adverse gastrointestinal effects when compared to commonly used painkillers such as ibuprofen. A marketing and promotion effort capitalized on these publications; Vioxx™ was the most heavily advertised prescription drug in 2000, and Celebrex™ was in seventh place.

Prostacyclin, a prostaglandin produced by COX-2 in blood vessel walls, opens blood vessels and prevents platelets from clumping. One theory is that when COX-2 is blocked, prostacyclin may also be suppressed, allowing platelets to stick together and causing blood vessels to constrict, which can lead to heart attacks and strokes. On September 27, 2004, Vioxx™ was voluntarily withdrawn from the market due to an increased risk of myocardial infarction (heart attack) and stroke, the principal outcomes of cardiovascular disease. At present, it is unclear whether this side effect also pertains to other drugs of this group or is specific to Vioxx™.

The risks associated with NSAID COX-2 inhibitors were discussed at an FDA meeting in February 2005. Speakers from public agencies, companies, and academia presented their findings. As a result of these findings, the FDA considered implementing changes in regulations. The manner in which the information was framed and communicated resulted in different and con-flicting interpretations of the data.[7]

Vioxx™ Risk Characterization Theater (RCT)

In order to determine the increased risk of cardiovascular events to indi-viduals taking the NSAID Vioxx™, we will apply the principles and approach used throughout this book.

- First, we calculate the absolute risk (AR) of cardiovascular events for individuals taking Vioxx™.
- Next, we calculate the AR of cardiovascular events for individuals who have not taken Vioxx™ (control group).
- Then, we find the absolute risk reduction (ARR) by comparing the difference in AR between these two groups.
- Finally, we present the results in the RCT.

The nine-month VIGOR study looked at 1,287 patients on Vioxx™ and 1,299 patients on a placebo. In the Vioxx™ group, there were 45 cardiovascular events, and in the control group taking the placebo there were 25 cardiovascular events. Therefore the AR in the Vioxx™ group was 3.5% (45/1,287), while the AR in the control group was 1.9% (25/1,299). The difference of 1.6% is the ARR.

Our 1,000 seat risk characterization theater (RCT) is filled with individuals taking Vioxx™. Over a nine-month period, 16 additional indi-viduals would experience a cardiovascular event, when compared to 1,000 individuals not taking this pain reliever. These individuals are represented by darkened seats in Fig. 6.1.

If you were considering taking Vioxx™ (assuming it was on the market) to relieve acute pain, or to relieve long-term pain associated with arthritis, you would have to determine whether this increased risk was acceptable to you. The uncertainty inherent in the VIGOR study was not quantified or reported, so you wouldn't know how precise the increased risk was: if the study were repeated, surely the number of heart attacks would not have been exactly the same. But regardless of this uncertainty, there is clearly a higher risk of a cardiovascular event if you are taking Vioxx™. You would

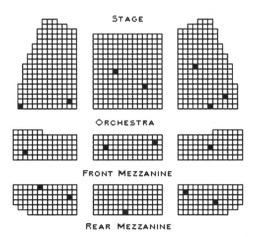

Fig. 6.1. The sixteen darkened seats in the Vioxx^{TM} RCT represent the number of additional people experiencing cardiovascular events when taking Vioxx^{TM} as compared to 1,000 individuals not taking this pain reliever over a 9-month period

need to assess the potential benefits of the drug for pain relief against the odds of an adverse effect, as reflected by the number of darkened seats in the Vioxx^{TM} RCT. Most likely, you would want to discuss this matter with your doctor, family, and others whose opinions you respect. But scientific and medical evidence wouldn't be able to tell you whether or not you should take Vioxx^{TM}; the final decision must be based on a value judgment and your level of acceptable risk.

7. Prostate Cancer Screening

The benefit of screening for prostate cancer using prostate-specific antigen (PSA) testing and digital rectal examination (DRE) is uncertain and is under evaluation in a randomized prospective trial [...]

G.L. Andriole et al.[1]

Issue

According to the National Cancer Institute (NCI), prostate cancer is the second leading cancer killer among men.[2] An estimated one in six men will be diagnosed with prostate cancer in his lifetime, and more than 30,000 Americans die of the disease each year. As a result, the NCI and other national medical organizations emphasize the need for routine screening for prostate cancer in men over the age of fifty.

Screening tests look for disease in people who don't have symptoms yet. Finding disease early can make treatment more effective, reduce suffering, and even prevent more serious problems. Screening has to be worth it: the occurrence of the disease and the chance of death must justify the effort and expense of screening.[3] Clearly, prostate cancer is common enough and serious enough to justify screening.

The prostate screening test has several components. It generally involves a digital rectal exam (DRE) and a blood test. If cancer is suspected, there is also a biopsy of prostate tissue. For healthy men over fifty, the American Cancer Society recommends an annual DRE and blood test.[1] The blood test measures levels of a protein produced in the prostate gland called prostate-specific antigen (PSA). Approximately 50% of "older men" now undergo routine PSA screenings.

The key question: *is there evidence that PSA screening alone increases survival by detecting prostate cancer early?* In other words, just how worthwhile is this PSA test? To answer this key question we need to determine the absolute risk reduction (ARR) for men who have had the screening test compared to men who have not.

Background

There is no such thing as a normal or even abnormal PSA level. But the more PSA in his blood, the more likely it is that a man has prostate cancer. Since PSA is produced in the body and can be measured as an indicator of prostate cancer, it is sometimes called a biomarker.

PSA test results are usually reported as nanograms of PSA per milliliter of blood, abbreviated ng/ml. A nanogram is a miniscule quantity; there are about 30 billion nanograms in a single ounce! A milliliter is about 15 drops. Many doctors are now using the following ranges and descriptors for blood PSA levels, with some variation:[4]

- 0-2.5 ng/ml is low
- 2.6-10 ng/ml is slightly to moderately elevated
- 10-19.9 ng/ml is moderately elevated
- 20 ng/ml or more is significantly elevated

Several factors can cause PSA levels to fluctuate, so a single elevated PSA test doesn't necessarily mean anything is wrong. The high test result could be due to a harmless enlargement of the prostate, an inflammation, an infection, or even age or race. So even though elevated PSA is a biomarker for prostate cancer, elevated levels don't necessarily mean that there is a problem.

Even if screening finds a tumor, the benefits aren't always clear-cut. Detecting a small tumor does not necessarily reduce your chance of dying from prostate cancer. Sometimes, PSA testing finds slow-growing, indolent tumors that are unlikely to be life threatening. If and when an annual PSA test finds a fast-growing tumor, it may be too late if the aggressive cancer has already spread to other parts of the body.[5]

Much is still unknown about prostate cancer. The causes aren't clear. The progression of the disease from initial symptoms to death isn't well-defined.[5] It seems some tumors are relatively inactive, while others progress rapidly.

Prostate cancer may even be two different diseases, a faster growing one and a slower growing one.

For the slow-growing cancer, the time from development of the disease to the onset of symptoms is drawn-out. This long period leaves ample time to detect the indolent cancer with a screening test. But symptoms appear early in the fast-growing form, and death often follows shortly. In these cases, the asymptomatic stage may not be long enough to allow detection by screening. And once symptoms are evident, you know you have the disease, so there's no point in screening to look for it.

There is also a problem with false positive and false negative screening test results. False positives can occur when the PSA level is elevated even though no cancer is present. Fortunately, most men with elevated PSA don't have cancer. Of course it's a big relief to find out that you don't have cancer after all. But the additional tests that prove the "positive" to be false have risks and cost money, not to mention the anxiety of waiting for results.[6] On the other hand, false negatives occur when prostate cancer hides behind an ordinary PSA level. Most prostate cancers are slow-growing and may exist for decades before they are large enough to cause symptoms. With a false negative, PSA results don't alert you to the problem even when the disease is progressing significantly.

PSA is just an indicator; a biopsy is needed to determine if prostate cancer is actually present. The more tissue removed during the biopsy, the greater the chance of detecting cancer. Biopsies can have side effects, including bleeding and infection. If a biopsy confirms cancer, the surgery to remove the tumor can cause incontinence (inability to control urine) and erectile dysfunction.[5]

Reports in the news suggest that prostate cancer is often a potent, fatal disease in fifty-year-old men. In fact, disease and death from prostate cancer are principally problems of older men. Age is the most common risk factor, with nearly 70% of prostate cancer cases occurring in men aged 65 and older.[7]

So what is the bottom line? As it turns out, researchers have found that extensive biopsies don't necessarily lead to a survival benefit due to early cancer detection.[8] This is primarily because prostate cancers detected during screening and biopsy are often indolent tumors. Men often choose surgery to remove these cancers. But even if they hadn't had surgery, men with this slow-growing form of the disease would likely have died of heart disease, diabetes, or another form of cancer before they even developed symptoms from the prostate tumor.

The current push for prostate cancer screening has increased identification and treatment of the disease. But even without treatment, many of these prostate cancer cases would still have been extremely low-risk. And the treatments themselves involve possible negative outcomes, as mentioned above. As a result, it is extremely difficult to determine the overall benefits, if any, of prostate screening.

Prostate Cancer Screening - Risk Characterization Theater (RCT)

At present, data are insufficient to calculate the absolute risk (AR) for individuals who were or were not screened. As a result, we cannot find the absolute risk reduction (ARR) for screening, and we cannot compare survival benefits between the two groups. Therefore it is not possible to construct a Prostate Cancer Screening RCT (Fig. 7.1, additional discussion in Chaps. 17 and 18).

What does all this mean? Let's go back to the key question. Is there evidence that prostate cancer screening leads to a survival benefit due to early detection of prostate cancer? The answer is no. There is no hard evidence, only anecdotal evidence. It's possible there is a benefit, but it's also possible that screening is without any value. The data are simply insufficient to answer the question with any degree of certainty.

Considering the uncertainty, the decision to have a prostate biopsy or surgery should be weighed carefully. The fact that we cannot calculate the ARR calls widespread PSA screening into question. It is possible that biopsies and surgery may not be warranted in some cases.

We do not mean to suggest that prostate cancer is not a deadly disease; thousands of men die from prostate cancer every year. What this case study does reveal, however, is the absence of evidence that screening tests reduce the risk of dying of this cancer. You may be willing to accept a

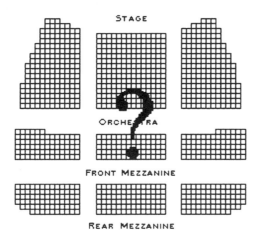

Fig. 7.1. There is insufficient information at this time to represent cancer risk reduction from prostate screening tests in an RCT

certain level of risk from biopsies or surgery, but there is no proof that you stand to benefit.

8. Elevated Cholesterol: A Primary Risk Factor for Heart Disease?

People whose blood cholesterol is low develop just as many plaques in their blood vessels as people whose cholesterol is high.

Uffe Ravnskov[1]

Issue

Coronary heart disease (CHD) is the leading cause of death in industrialized countries throughout the world, and is by far the number one killer in the United States. Over 70 million Americans have some form of cardiovascular disease, and approximately one million of them die from it each year. Heart disease accounted for nearly 40% of all deaths in the United States at the turn of the 21st century.[2]

These are frightening statistics. So it is not surprising that CHD has attracted intense interest in the public health community for decades. With "baby boomers" aging and more individuals being affected by CHD, this interest will continue to grow. It's increasingly important that we understand CHD so we can reduce or eliminate those conditions responsible for this disease. Unfortunately, in spite of years of research and costly clinical and epidemiological studies targeting CHD, scientists and physicians have not been able to discover any definitive cause and effect relationships.

The causes of CHD and of its precursor, atherosclerosis – in which fatty deposits, cholesterol, cellular waste products, calcium, and other substances build up on the lining of arteries – are still unknown. So judgments about why CHD occurs and how to control it are based on the presence or absence of risk factors. There are many risk factors which have been associated with atherosclerosis and CHD. At present, the list includes: cigarette smoking, elevated blood pressure, elevated cholesterol, low serum HDL cholesterol, diabetes, advancing age, obesity, abdominal obesity, physical inactivity, family history of premature coronary heart disease, ethnic characteristics, psychosocial factors, elevated serum triglycerides, small LDL particles, elevated serum homocysteine, elevated serum lipoprotein(a), elevated fibrinogen, elevated inflammatory markers... and the list of suspect factors goes on. Yet most of these risk factors individually have almost no value in predicting whether CHD or atherosclerosis will occur.

The prevailing view is that elevated blood serum cholesterol is the primary controllable risk factor (as opposed to uncontrollable risk factors, such as age and genetics) in the development of atherosclerosis and CHD. Reports in the media state rather convincingly that the risk of CHD is markedly lower when blood serum cholesterol levels are lowered; the current benchmark falls in the vicinity of 200 mg/100mL or less. It is also assumed that lowering cholesterol dramatically reduces the risk of suffering from atherosclerosis and CHD. As a result, approximately 200 million Americans currently undergo cholesterol screening tests, 13 million are on cholesterol-lowering drugs, and 52 million are on cholesterol-lowering diets. In the Third Report of the National Cholesterol Education Program, a government-sponsored panel recently suggested that the number of Americans taking cholesterol-lowering drugs be raised to approximately 36 million, and that more Americans – about 65 million – should be on cholesterol-lowering diets.[3]

But, as is usually the case when risk factors are involved, the relationship between cholesterol levels and the incidence of CHD is not as clear as popular reports suggest. A doctor at the Harvard Medical School notes that "[h]alf of all myocardial infarctions [heart attacks] and strokes occur in individuals without elevated cholesterol levels ...."[4] In a recent article, cardiovascular pioneer Dr. Michael DeBakey found that elevated cholesterol levels had no effect on the recurrence of coronary disease.[5]

Doctors have admitted the difficulties of diagnosis from cholesterol levels alone. Dr. William Kannel, one of the first directors of the famous clinical Framingham Study on the relationship of cholesterol levels and CHD, stated that "diagnosis of overt heart disease on the basis of lipid [cholesterol] levels alone is simply not feasible."[6] Dr. William Castelli, another former director of the Framingham study, wrote, "Obviously, the total cholesterol value cannot accurately predict which patients have a [...] problem when the cholesterol levels are between 200 and 250 mg or even between 150 and 250 mg."[7]

Dr. Mark Hegsted, former director of the US Department of Agriculture Human Nutrition Center, observed that the report of the World Health Organization and many others have emphasized how the majority of heart attacks apparently occur in individuals with serum cholesterol levels below 240 mg.[8] In 1989, Dr. Castelli reported that "one-half of all heart attacks now occur in people whose serum cholesterol level is 225 mg or less."[9] Since the average cholesterol level among adult Americans is about 220 mg, his statement means that heart attacks occur almost equally among people with normal and elevated cholesterol levels.

So we have a conundrum. Does lowering cholesterol result in a marked reduction in the incidence of CHD? Or, is it impossible to predict with any degree of certainty whether there is a difference in the incidence of CHD in populations with elevated and normal cholesterol levels? Cholesterol can be designated a primary risk factor for CHD only if individuals with elevated blood serum cholesterol levels have an appreciably higher incidence of atherosclerosis and CHD than individuals with normal cholesterol levels. Looking at it another way, if individuals with normal and elevated blood serum cholesterol have essentially the same incidence of CHD, then an elevated level of cholesterol in the blood cannot be identified as a primary risk factor.

A key question arises. *Within a population, do individuals with essentially normal blood serum cholesterol have a lower incidence of coronary heart disease than individuals with elevated levels of blood serum cholesterol?*

Background

The rationale for the focus on cholesterol as a risk factor is best illustrated by a recent advertisement for a popular cholesterol-lowering statin drug, asserting cholesterol's role in the development of CHD. The ad states that plaque forms when too much LDL (bad) cholesterol builds up on the inside of your arteries. It also points out that this buildup of plaque causes the arteries to become thicker, harder, and less flexible – thereby restricting blood flow, which can cause a heart attack or a stroke. Since cholesterol and other components found in plaque are, in large part, responsible for atherosclerosis and CHD, it seems reasonable to assume that lowering the level of blood serum cholesterol – the cholesterol in the bloodstream – will reduce the incidence of these diseases. It would be counterintuitive to come to any other conclusion.

While the quoted advertisement is accurate when it states that cholesterol builds up in arteries and statins reduce blood cholesterol levels, it does not implicate *elevated* blood cholesterol levels in the development of atherosclerosis and CHD. For example, individuals with *normal* cholesterol levels may also have arteries with plaque buildup (i.e., blood serum cholesterol levels may have no correlation with the prevalence and incidence of plaque in arteries). Indeed, the opening statement by Dr. Ravnskov indicates that people with low and high cholesterol have the same number of plaques in their arteries.[1] It would be important, therefore, to determine the difference in absolute risk between these two populations. Published clinical studies shed light on the subject and provide the data needed to evaluate the risks associated with different blood serum cholesterol levels.

The best-known clinical study attempting to correlate blood serum cholesterol levels and the incidence of CHD is the Framingham Study. This study, which began in 1948, was supported by the National Heart, Lung, and Blood Institute and involved some 5,000 men and women from a Boston suburb. These individuals were followed and examined for over 50 years to determine if there was an association between serum blood cholesterol levels and CHD.[6]

In 1979, an article titled "Cholesterol in the Prediction of Atherosclerotic Disease – New Perspectives Based on the Framingham Study" concluded that "prospective data at Framingham and elsewhere have shown conclusively that risk of coronary heart disease in persons younger than age 50 is strikingly related to the serum total cholesterol level."[10] That is strong language. But the data didn't support this confident assertion. Though the article was widely quoted and reinforced the prevailing views regarding cholesterol and CHD, it contained a graph that shows that nearly the same number of individuals with essentially normal and elevated cholesterol died of CHD (the graph is presented in Appendix B).

The serum cholesterol level of 220 mg per 100 ml – frequently abbreviated to "220 mg" in everyday speech – is the line between essentially normal and elevated (please note that this chapter adopts the abbreviated notation). However, this is a moving target, and the number for essentially normal has been going down lately. In the Framingham data, the group of men with blood serum cholesterol levels above 220 mg died at about the same rate as the men with cholesterol levels below 220 mg.

The largest and most comprehensive clinical study on cholesterol levels and heart disease is the Multiple Risk Factor Intervention Trial, or MRFIT.[11,12] In this study, over 350,000 male participants had their cholesterol levels measured and monitored for 6 years. The blood serum cholesterol level at which 50% of the population died from CHD virtually duplicated the results obtained from the Framingham study (in the case of MRFIT, the 50% level was 225 mg; see Appendix B).

These two large clinical studies, which are the most often cited, have shown that nearly the same number of individuals with normal and elevated cholesterol have atherosclerosis and CHD. But what does "nearly the same" mean? How can we determine if we should be screened for blood serum cholesterol levels, eat cholesterol free food, and take drugs to lower our cholesterol levels?

Risk Characterization

Using the MRFIT[12] data, Fig. 8.1 shows the annual number of CHD deaths per thousand individuals at different serum cholesterol levels.

The graph shows annual CHD deaths per thousand individuals increasing by 1/1,000 (a rate of 0.1%) as the cholesterol level climbs from 150 to 250 mg. Portions of the above data set can be visualized using our Risk Characterization Theater (RCT) graphic. The first Cholesterol RCT in Fig. 8.2 represents 1,000 people whose mean total blood serum cholesterol level is 280 mg – a level uniformly characterized as significantly elevated. The one darkened seat represents the single individual at increased risk of death from CHD when compared to 1,000 individuals with an essentially normal cholesterol level (between 210 and 220 mg).

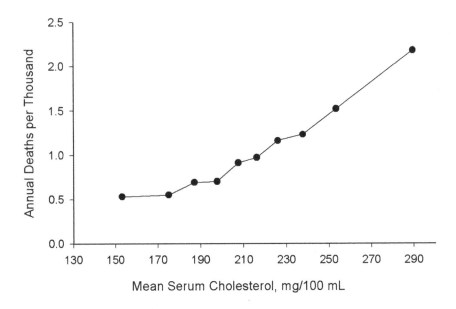

Fig. 8.1. Annual CHD deaths per 1,000 individuals as a function of serum cholesterol levels, based on data from the MRFIT study[12]

Our second example (Fig. 8.3) involves two RCTs that represent 2,000 people whose mean total blood serum cholesterol level is 250 mg – a far more representative level, also uniformly characterized as significantly elevated. In this instance, there is one darkened seat representing the single individual at increased annual risk of dying from a heart attack when compared to 2,000 individuals with an essentially normal cholesterol level (between 210 and 220 mg).

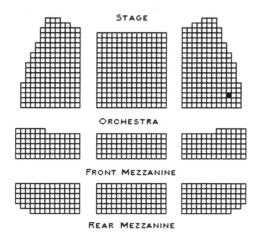

Fig. 8.2. Out of 1,000 people with a significantly elevated cholesterol level of 280 mg, there will be one additional death per year from CHD (represented by a single darkened seat) as compared to 1,000 people with essentially normal cholesterol (between 210 and 220 mg)

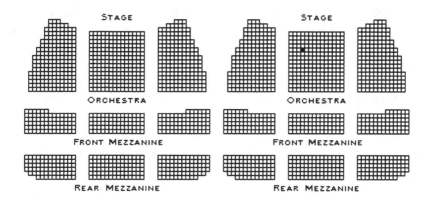

Fig. 8.3. Out of 2,000 people with a significantly elevated cholesterol level of 250 mg, there will be one additional death per year from CHD (represented by a single darkened seat) as compared to 2,000 people with essentially normal cholesterol (between 210 and 220 mg)

A third RCT graphic (Fig. 8.4) compares the difference in annual deaths per 1,000 for the group with less than 210 mg cholesterol to the group with cholesterol between 210 and 250 mg. The average annual death rate for the group with essentially normal cholesterol is about 0.75 per 1,000 people. The average for the group with elevated cholesterol is about 1.25 deaths per 1,000 each year. The difference is 0.5 deaths per 1,000 people, which is the same as one death per 2,000 people each year. For the RCT graphic in this example, there is one darkened seat representing the increased annual risk for 2,000 individuals with cholesterol between 210 to 250 mg when compared to 2,000 individuals with blood serum cholesterol less than 210 mg.

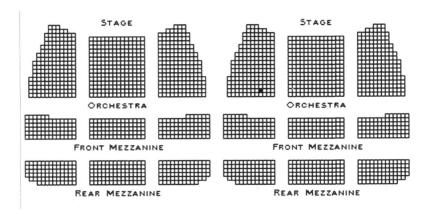

Fig. 8.4. Out of 2,000 people with a cholesterol level between 210 and 250 mg, there will be one additional death each year from CHD (represented by a single darkened seat) as compared to 2,000 people with cholesterol lower than 210 mg

It should be emphasized that there is uncertainty in these numbers. For example, one reason for the gradual increase in annual CHD deaths per 1,000 individuals through the entire range of blood serum cholesterol levels is that both cholesterol levels and the incidence of CHD increase with age. It's hard to adjust data to account for these variables. Another possible reason is that CHD deaths at the higher end of the cholesterol levels shown in Fig. 8.1 – associated with about 5% of the population – are likely to include individuals with diabetes, a genetic disorder (familial hypercholesteremia), and other diseases. People with these diseases have a higher risk of dying from CHD but apparently were not excluded from the analysis.

While it's hard to quantify the uncertainty in these numbers, these values were obtained from very large clinical studies and probably are a good estimate of reality. The Cholesterol RCTs provide a "ballpark" estimate of the individual risk due to elevated blood serum cholesterol levels. If you excluded the 5% of the population with genetic disorders, diabetes, etc., then the apparent difference between populations with high and low cholesterol levels would in all likelihood be less pronounced.

But let's assume for a moment that Fig. 8.1 is correct. Let's say the gentle upward trend from the lowest to the highest cholesterol level is legitimate. Let's forget about difficulties in excluding diabetics and people with genetic abnormalities, and in normalizing for age and unknown additive or synergistic effects of multiple risk factors. Then in a group of 1,000 individuals with elevated cholesterol, there will be approximately 1 additional death annually when compared to 1,000 individuals with normal cholesterol. Therefore, 99.9% of the individuals with elevated cholesterol would not be affected.

You would then have to ask yourself whether an annual risk of 1 in 1,000 (0.1%) constitutes an acceptable risk? Is a 0.1% risk reduction worth modifying your diet, changing major elements of your lifestyle, and taking expensive drugs (see Chap. 9 on statins) in an attempt to lower your cholesterol to essentially normal levels or below? You will need to think long and hard about your level of acceptable risk and what course of action to take. Another way to look at these results would be to say that for 999 out of 1,000 individuals each year, it makes no difference whether they have elevated cholesterol or normal cholesterol in terms of whether or not they develop CHD.

Individual Risk vs. Nationwide Risk

Some people may conclude that a 0.1% risk is not worth taking; these individuals will probably be concerned and take action to reduce blood serum cholesterol levels. But others might question whether the increase in the level of risk associated with elevated cholesterol is serious enough to warrant concern.

We might also wonder why these data seem to fly in the face of reports from physicians, drug companies, and government agencies. Why would medical practitioners, agencies like the FDA, and pharmaceutical companies misrepresent the truth? But the answer is not that they are pulling the wool over our eyes. It's just that they are presenting results that relate to nationwide health risks instead of individual risks. They also have their own interests and motives and tend to characterize data in a way that supports their own particular views and perspectives – a trait that we all seem to possess in one form or another.

For example, drug companies almost always use relative numbers to explain the benefits of drugs to reduce cholesterol. This is a valid statistical approach. It is not a misrepresentation of data, but it does makes the benefits from these drugs seem dramatic and, at the same time, distort the risks associated with elevated cholesterol.

Federal agencies and physicians focus on health benefits to the entire nation rather than to the individual. So if there are approximately 50 million Americans with elevated cholesterol, and if CHD risks for those people are 0.1% higher than for individuals with normal cholesterol, then 50,000 lives might be saved annually by lowering those people's cholesterol levels. Risks are presented in the context of national impacts in much the same way as the EPA communicates risks from exposure to dioxin, lead, mercury, and other environmental contaminants.

As this book has mentioned before, it is virtually impossible for us to visualize or relate to risks and benefits to millions of people. When information is presented that way, it is certainly hard for us each to imagine our own personal risk or benefit. Unfortunately, very little effort has been made to provide data in a format (e.g., RCTs) that could help citizens participate in critical health decisions. Public and private health institutions agree that individuals should be involved in decisions about medical intervention and health risk analysis. While this may be an oft-repeated objective, the public still doesn't have ready access to data that would empower each of us to base our personal decisions on the level of individual risk that feels acceptable.

9. Statins, Cholesterol, and Coronary Heart Disease

If the major benefits of statins are mediated through their effects on inflammation, thrombosis, and oxidation, we would also expect the relative benefits of statin therapy to be independent of baseline LDL cholesterol level.

R.A. Haywood et al.[1]

Issue

Statins – Lescol™, Lipitor™, Mevacor™, Pravacol™, and Zocor™ – are the most widely used prescription drugs in the world. Over 20 million people worldwide take statins, and the resulting annual sales exceeded 16 billion dollars in 2001.[2] Why are they so popular? People take statins to lower their cholesterol. Indeed, these drugs can reduce blood serum cholesterol levels by 30 to 40% or more.[2]

As described in the previous chapter, experts have found that the incidence of coronary heart disease (CHD) is essentially the same for people with elevated and normal blood serum cholesterol levels. The Cholesterol Risk Characterization Theaters (RCTs) shown in Chap. 8 suggest that the level of benefit from reducing cholesterol levels may not support the contention that cholesterol is a primary risk factor for CHD.

Yet many of the people who take statins to lower their cholesterol do so in the hopes of reducing their risk of heart disease. Two key questions arise. *Do individuals taking statins have a lower incidence of CHD when compared to individuals not taking these drugs? If so, are the benefits due to lowering blood serum cholesterol levels, or are they due to something else?*

In 2004, a National Cholesterol Education Program (NCEP) panel of experts stated that consistent and compelling evidence showed a strong relationship between LDL cholesterol levels (so-called "bad" cholesterol) and cardiovascular risks.[3,4] The panel recommended that physicians try to reduce LDL cholesterol to less than 70 mg/100 ml in patients at very high risk for cardiovascular events[3,4]

In a more recent article (Oct. 2006) in the Annals of Internal Medicine, the connection between LDL and heart disease wasn't quite so strong. The authors found no evidence that individuals with LDL cholesterol levels below 130 mg/100 ml would benefit from further reducing their blood serum cholesterol. And yet, the authors conclude, "there is clear and compelling evidence that most patients at high risk for cardiovascular disease should be taking at least a moderate dose of a statin if tolerated, *even if their natural LDL cholesterol level is low*" [emphasis added].[1] How can this be? The apparent contradiction would be resolved if statins were active by some other mechanism besides lowering cholesterol. The authors based their conclusions on a comprehensive review and analysis of what has been published on the topic.

So what's the bottom line? Statins are certainly effective at reducing cholesterol levels. Doctors and researchers generally agree that statins also lower the incidence of CHD. However, it's not clear whether statins' heart benefits come from lowering cholesterol or from something else they do in the body. On the other hand, does it really matter why statins work? Maybe cholesterol levels are relevant, maybe not – but so what? If statins reduce the incidence of CHD, shouldn't everyone take them? After all, heart attacks are often deadly.

However, many of us aren't going to die of a heart attack, or even experience CHD symptoms. Some of us have elevated cholesterol but no other risk factors for cardiovascular disease. Should we endure the cost and possible adverse effects of statins? Should we take a combination of drugs to continue to lower our blood serum cholesterol levels? What about swearing off tasty foods that are high in cholesterol? These are legitimate questions in spite of the continued focus on reducing cholesterol levels. Currently, opinions vary in the medical and scientific communities on the merits of prescribing statins to low risk populations.[5,6]

Before taking statins (or any drug for that matter), it is smart to do a little fact-finding. We must determine what these potent drugs do, what they don't do, and for whom. After all, even if they have great benefits for some people, there's still no "free lunch"! Statins can cause side-effects and complications like rhabdomyolysis (muscle destruction); abnormal changes in liver function; myopathy; adverse changes to memory, thinking, and concentration; depression and irritability; increased pain, tingling, and numbness; sleep problems; sexual dysfunction; blood sugar changes; and nausea. Some of these side effects can affect a significant number of people. For example, nine out of every hundred people in clinical trials complained that statins affected their digestive system, while only four out of every hundred complained when they were given a placebo.[7,8]

Background

Cholesterol is essential for life, and so we "build" cholesterol in our bodies. Statins, on the other hand, reduce cholesterol levels. The method or "mechanism" by which they act has been verified in a number of studies:[9] statins prevent a specific enzyme (HMG-CoA reductase) from functioning properly. This enzyme is an important worker on the cholesterol assembly line. Stopping the enzyme from doing its job ultimately prevents the body from making enough cholesterol.

Since the body requires cholesterol to function properly, there needs to be some way to compensate for the cholesterol "shortage" when statins interfere with the assembly line. Our cells need to get cholesterol from somewhere else. One easy source is the cholesterol in our blood.

So statins have another effect. They also cause changes that let cells absorb cholesterol from the blood stream better. Taking statins leads to an increase in the number of cholesterol receptors on the surface of our cells.[9] These receptors are like microscopic doors that allow cholesterol to cross from the blood into the cell. More doors means more cholesterol can enter the cell. Once inside, cholesterol can perform its many necessary functions. To summarize, statins make cells sponge up the cholesterol they need from the blood, instead of building it themselves. This lowers blood serum cholesterol levels.

It looks like statins do many additional things in the body besides decreasing LDL cholesterol levels.[10,11] Some of these effects are listed in Box 9.1. Notice in particular that statins may play a role in reducing inflammation and blood clots. Indeed, the cardiovascular benefits of statin therapy may come from these effects on inflammation and clot formation.[12] Statins can affect the innermost layer of cells lining our arteries (the endothelium), make smooth muscle cells less active, control inflammation, and affect the physiology of the artery wall.[13] These changes have been associated with limiting the development of atherosclerosis, which is the precursor or gateway disease to cardiovascular disease (CVD). It is possible that one or more of these mechanisms of action is responsible for the reduced incidence of CVD following statin use. Note that at times the terms cardiovascular disease and coronary heart disease are both used when describing the benefits of statins. CVD is a general diagnostic category consisting of several separate diseases of the heart and circulatory system, including CHD and stroke. Throughout this chapter, the terms CHD and CVD will be used consistently with how each clinical study reported its results.

Box 9.1. These effects have been reported to have molecular mechanisms that are independent of statins' effect on low-density lipoprotein cholesterol.
Known Lipid Independent Effects of Statins (adapted from ref. 1)
Increased synthesis of nitric oxide
Inhibition of free radical release
Decreased synthesis of endothelin-1
Inhibition of low-density lipoprotein cholesterol oxidation
Up-regulation of endothelial progenitor cells
Reduced number and activity of inflammatory cells
Reduced level of C-reactive protein
Reduced macrophage cholesterol accumulation
Reduced production of metalloproteinases
Inhibition of platelet adhesion or aggregation
Reduced fibrinogen concentration
Reduced blood viscosity

Some statin trials don't line up well with the hypothesis that lowering LDL cholesterol reduces CVD. For example, trials have found that statins substantially reduce the risk of stroke. This benefit is consistent with these drugs' reported ability to reduce the formation of clots in blood vessels. However, the stroke benefit may not have much to do with the LDL-lowering effects of statins, since elevated LDL levels are not a major independent risk factor for stroke.[14] Furthermore, a large statin trial conducted in dialysis patients found no substantial cardiovascular benefit, despite 42% reductions in LDL cholesterol levels.[15] These results suggest that even meaningful reductions in LDL are not always associated with clinically significant decreases in cardiovascular risk.

Indeed, if statins' primary benefits are a result of mechanisms unrelated to lowering LDL cholesterol levels, then we should focus more on the other risk factors for CVD. More resources should be allocated to clarify which conditions put people at the greatest risk for heart disease, and whether statins are effective against these conditions. Since our understanding is still incomplete, it is possible that millions of people are taking statins who shouldn't be, and millions of people who should be aren't. If cholesterol is not the primary risk factor for CHD, then some people are unnecessarily bearing the cost and potential side effects of cholesterol-reducing drugs. But if statins are effective against something other than cholesterol, then individuals who could potentially benefit from taking statins are being overlooked.

Risk Characterization

A number of large, controlled, clinical trials with statins have been conducted involving tens of thousands of people. These clinical trails have included people without a history of CVD who take statins for "primary prevention," as well as individuals with a history of CVD who take statins for "secondary prevention." Results from these studies show that statins do reduce the incidence of cardiovascular events for both groups.[16]

Diabetes, age, high blood pressure, smoking, family history, and even gender can all play a role in CVD, so these characteristics are called "risk factors." Many study participants have not one but multiple risk factors for CVD. But the risk factors vary from study to study, which makes it difficult to come to any meaningful conclusions about which patients will benefit from taking one or more specific statin drug. Maybe people with diabetes will respond better to one drug, while smokers with high blood pressure will respond better to a different one, but researchers just don't have enough information to know yet. In other words, the uncertainty surrounding statin use remains high. However, one thing is clear: people who have already had a heart attack benefit more from statins than people with no history of CVD.

Information in the Statin RCTs that appear in this section came from a summary[16] that examined and compared the results of seven different studies. Four of them were major studies about the use of three statins (Zocor™, Lipitor™, and Pravacol™) by people without previous CVD. The other three studies investigated the use of the same three statins in populations with previous CVD. All of these clinical studies were conducted over the last decade or so, involved thousands of individuals with different sets of risk factors, lasted approximately 5 years, and provided data to calculate the cardiovascular benefits.

While the results can certainly be interpreted in a variety of ways, they give a sense of the overall benefits from taking the three statins studied. The Statin RCTs presented below show the number of patients who benefited by taking statins for five years. The benefit was a decrease in cardiovascular events – generally heart attack or CHD death, depending on the study.[16]

Primary Prevention Studies

The Statin RCTs shown in Fig. 9.1 represent individuals without previous CVD who have taken Zocor™, Lipitor™, or Pravacol™. The people who took statins experienced fewer cardiovascular events in comparison to the people who did not take statins. The darkened seats in each example represent the number of individuals without previous CVD who benefited from statin use, compared to people who didn't take statins.

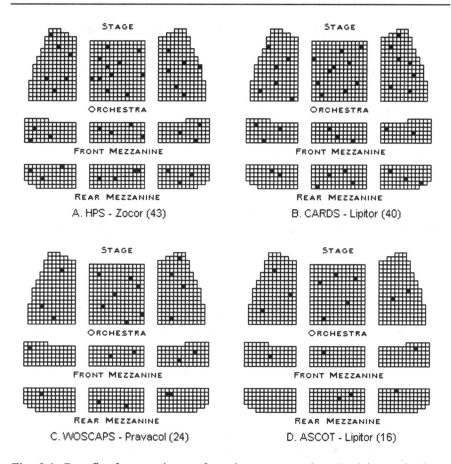

Fig. 9.1. Benefits from statin use for primary prevention. Participants in these studies did not have previous cardiovascular disease. The darkened seats in each RCT represent the number of individuals out of 1,000 who avoided CVD over a five-year period by taking statins, as compared to people who didn't take statins. **A.** *Heart Protection Study Group* (HPS) participants took Zocor^{TM} (Simvastatin) and saw an absolute benefit of 43 per thousand; **B.** *Collaborative Atorvastatin Diabetes Study* (CARDS) participants took Lipitor^{TM} (Atorvastatin) and saw an absolute benefit of 40 per thousand; **C.** *West of Scotland Coronary Prevention Study* (WOSCAPS) participants took Pravacol^{TM} (Pravastatin) and saw an absolute benefit of 24 per thousand; and **D.** *Anglo-Scandinavian Cardiac Outcomes Trial* (ASCOT) participants took Lipitor^{TM} (Atorvastatin) and saw an absolute benefit of 16 per thousand

In summary, between 16 and 43 out of 1,000 individuals without previous CVD benefited from taking statins over a five-year period when compared to individuals not taking these drugs in the primary prevention studies. The average of these studies is about 30, so approximately 30 out of 1,000 people benefited. In other words, the average absolute benefit rate for using the statins for primary prevention is about 3%. This means that the other 97% of people taking statins for primary prevention did not benefit from taking these drugs, at least in terms of CVD.

Secondary Prevention Studies

The Statin RCTs shown in Fig. 9.2 represent individuals with previous CVD who have taken Zocor[TM], Lipitor[TM], or Pravacol[TM]. The people who took statins experienced fewer cardiovascular events in comparison to the people who did not take the statins. The darkened seats in each example represent the number of people with previous CVD who benefited from statin use, compared to people not taking statins.

To summarize, for those people who had previous CVD, between 58 and 76 out of 1,000 individuals benefited from taking statins over a five-year period when compared to those who didn't take the drugs. The average of these studies is about 67, so approximately 67 out of 1,000 people benefited. In other words, the absolute benefit rate from using the statins for secondary prevention is almost 7%. Conversely, 93% of the individuals in the studies did not benefit from taking the statins. Comparing Figs. 9.1 and 9.2, the benefits to individuals with previous heart attacks are clearly greater than the benefits for individuals with no previous CVD.

Discussion

The results from these statin studies support the view that these drugs provide benefits greater than the benefits which would be achieved by lowering blood serum cholesterol levels. The data presented in the previous chapter show that every year, at most 1 person out of 1,000 avoids a fatal heart attack by lowering his or her cholesterol from significantly elevated to essentially normal. This means that 5 lives out of 1,000 might be saved over a five-year period. For individuals without previous CVD, the benefit of taking statins over five years is many times higher: on average, 30 out

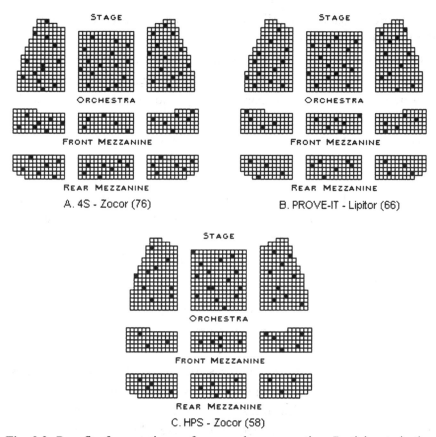

Fig. 9.2. Benefits from statin use for secondary prevention. Participants in these studies had previous cardiovascular disease. The darkened seats in each RCT represent the number of individuals out of 1,000 who avoided CVD over a five-year period by taking statins, as compared to people who didn't take statins. **A.** *Scandinavian Simvastatin Survival Study Group* (4S) participants took Zocor[TM] (Simvastatin) and saw an absolute benefit of 76 per thousand, **B.** *Pravastatin or Atorvastatin Evaluation and Infection Therapy* (PROVE-IT) participants took Lipitor[TM] (Atorvastatin) and saw an absolute benefit of 66 per thousand, and **C.** *Heart Protection Study* (HPS) participants took Zocor[TM] (Simvastatin) and saw an absolute benefit of 58 per thousand

of 1,000 experienced a benefit (Fig. 9.1). For those who already had CVD, the benefits of statins were even greater: on average, 67 out of 1,000 benefited (Fig. 9.2). The outcomes of the statin clinical trials support the idea that mechanisms other than the lowering of cholesterol (such as those in

Box 9.1) are probably primarily responsible for the reduced incidence of CVD following statin use.

These results are based on the absolute benefits from taking statins, as reported in clinical trials. The RCTs show the marginal increase in absolute benefit, calculated by comparing people who took the drug to people who didn't. For determining health benefits and risks, these absolute numbers are far more useful than relative values and percent changes. As described in previous chapters, relative values don't tell the whole story, so they tend to present a biased picture of the benefits and risks of intervention. Relative values are valid, but they're harder to interpret when we have to make a decision like whether or not to take a cholesterol-lowering drug. Unfortunately, it's hard to find much information about statins except relative numbers and percentage changes – unless you have access to data from scientific studies.

Individual vs. Nationwide Benefits

As mentioned in the chapter about cholesterol, nearly 70 million Americans have some form of CVD, and approximately one million die from it each year.[17] Based on the clinical trials shown in Fig. 9.2, about 7% of these individuals could potentially benefit if they were all to take statins. That's almost 5 million people! It's no wonder that statins are the best-selling prescription drug in the world. As impressive as these benefits appear, individual decisions shouldn't be based on nationwide benefit numbers.

Consider the population that falls in the category "without previous CVD." Since the population of the US is about 300 million, this group is considerably larger than the group "with previous CVD." As described above, about 3% of people in this group benefit from taking statins, and the other 97% don't benefit.

Imagine yourself in a hypothetical situation. You are one of the approximately 180 million adult Americans who don't have any previous CVD. You have just had your annual medical exam. Your doctor tells you that everything is fine except for your total blood serum cholesterol level, which is a bit high at 245 mg. Your physician recommends that you should start taking a statin to lower your cholesterol.

You already know a little about cholesterol. For people with your cholesterol level, you know that around 1 person out of 2,000 will benefit from lowering his or her cholesterol to a normal level. You also know that these data came from studies including older individuals and people with diabetes and other diseases. These are conditions and situations which raise the risk of CVD, but don't apply to you.

Imagine that from your perspective, your blood serum cholesterol level just doesn't warrant taking statins. In your mind, the possible benefits of lowering your cholesterol with statins don't justify the costs, risks, and lifestyle changes. However, as you understand it, statins could also have other benefits – benefits that may be more important than lowering cholesterol. Maybe these would tip the balance in favor of taking statins after all. So you ask your doctor about other risk factors you might have for heart disease (such as C-reactive protein). Will statins affect these risk factors? Will they lower your risk for CVD by means other than lowering LDL cholesterol levels?

So you get all the sound advice you can, you evaluate your situation, you assess the benefits, you think about how much risk you're willing to live with, and you proceed accordingly. The decision to begin taking any drug for an extended period of time is an important one and should be made after careful deliberation. This is particularly true for statins, since it's a bit cloudy how much the heart benefits are associated with lowering LDL cholesterol levels.

10. Colorectal Cancer Screening

Three randomized trials have demonstrated reduction in mortality from colorectal cancer (CRC) by repeated screening with faecal occult blood tests...

O.D. Jorgensen[1]

Issue

The American Cancer Society estimates that over 107,000 people were newly diagnosed with colon cancer in 2002. More than 56,000 people died of this cancer that same year.[2] Colorectal cancer develops in the rectum or the colon, and is one of the leading cancer killers in the US. Both men and women are at risk. Ninety-three percent of cases occur in people age 50 or older. The risk of developing colorectal cancer increases with age.[3]

There are screening programs for colorectal cancer. The primary purpose of a screening test is to identify disease in people who don't have symptoms yet. Catching the problem at an early stage may allow treatment to prevent the full-blown disease, or at least to reduce its severity. The occurrence of the disease and the mortality from the disease must justify the effort and the expense of screening.[4] In the case of colorectal cancer, these criteria have been met. The screening test looks for cancerous cells in the colon.

The key question: *is there evidence that colorectal cancer screening confers a survival benefit due to the early detection of colorectal cancer?* In other words, what is the absolute risk reduction (ARR) for people who have had the screening test compared to people who have not?

Background

There are a number of screening tests available for colorectal cancer. By far, the most significant data on benefits of colorectal cancer screening involve a combination of two specific tests: the fecal occult blood (FOB) test, followed by a colonoscopy if necessary. In this chapter, screening refers to the combination of these two tests.

The FOB test checks for blood hidden in the stool. Blood in a stool sample suggests the possibility of cancer. There are a number of other possibilities as well, so follow-up testing is usually recommended to identify the origin of the problem. In fact, a positive FOB result almost always leads to colonoscopy.

A colonoscopy is designed to determine the source of the bleeding and to look for injury. This screening test allows a doctor to examine the entire colon and the lining of the rectum using a thin, flexible, lighted tube called a colonoscope. The device is also used to find and remove polyps, which then are examined under a microscope by a pathologist to determine if they are cancerous. Colonoscopy is considered an invasive procedure. The patient is given an intravenous sedative beforehand. In rare cases, there are serious consequences such as hemorrhage, perforation of the bowel wall, and even death.

Risk Characterization

Three large studies were carried out in the US, the UK, and Denmark, starting in the 1970s. More than 335,000 subjects between the ages of 45 and 80 participated. Researchers collected follow-up data thirteen or more years later.[1,5,6,7] The data demonstrate a reduction in colorectal cancer mortality among those subjects who underwent FOB/colonoscopy screening, compared with those who didn't undergo the proposed screening tests.

From these studies, we can calculate that screening reduced lifetime colorectal cancer mortality from approximately 2.9 to 1.9 deaths for every 1,000 subject individuals. Screened individuals had an absolute risk (AR) of approximately 0.2% (1.9 / 1,000 ≈ 0.2%). Individuals not screened had an AR of approximately 0.3% (2.9 / 1,000 ≈ 0.3%). All these people were in the average risk category because they didn't have a family history of colorectal cancer. The absolute risk reduction (ARR) for these average individuals was 0.1% (0.3% - 0.2% = 0.1%) or 1/1,000 over a lifetime. In other words, 1,000 people were screened before a benefit to one person was observed. The number needed to treat (NNT) is 1,000.

How often do average people have to be screened in order to see this benefit? Researchers determined that you would need an FOB test at least once every 2 years from the age of 50 until the age of 75.[1] If the FOB test were ever positive, colonoscopy or another equivalent diagnostic test would be proposed.

Our Colorectal Cancer Screening RCT (Fig. 10.1) contains 1,000 individuals who were screened for colorectal cancer. The darkened seat represents the one life saved, compared to 1,000 individuals who did not undergo screening.

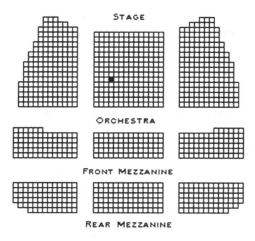

Fig. 10.1. Colorectal Cancer Screening RCT. There is one darkened seat to show that one colon cancer death will be avoided for every 1,000 people screened

As with any other risk-based decision, you need to assess the benefits from this screening test in the context of risks associated with intervention, costs, and inconvenience. Given the somewhat small ARR number (0.1%), the level of uncertainty is comparatively high. It's likely that you would want to discuss this matter with you doctor, family, and others. Your final decision on whether or not to sign up for a colorectal cancer screening program will be based primarily on your level of acceptable risk.

Individual Benefits vs. Nationwide Benefits

Epidemiological uncertainty aside, if all of the 335,000 people in the three studies mentioned above were screened using FOB/colonoscopy, there would be 335 fewer deaths from colorectal cancer (335,000 / 1,000 = 335). If the number of individuals being screened was expanded to include all the residents of the US (or any other country) between 45 and 80 years old, the number of lives saved would increase in proportion to the number of people screened.

Organizations concerned with public health issues want to reduce overall deaths nationwide (e.g., Centers for Disease Control, American Cancer Society, National Institutes of Health). As public health stewards, researchers, and advocates, these groups report country-wide statistics on cancer and other diseases. Nationwide death benefits from colon cancer screening can be in the thousands. Reducing colon cancer deaths is certainly a laudable objective. But nationwide numbers are not particularly useful for individuals who are trying to understand their individual level of risk and decide if it's acceptable to them.

We need a more accessible framework, one that enables us to comprehend health benefits in a more relevant, direct, and practical context. Overall health benefits to thousands of individuals in a population of hundreds of millions are hard to imagine. They translate poorly, if at all, at the personal level. We need to be able to obtain and interpret data which will permit us to make a decision based on our own level of acceptable risk (see Chap. 18 on Acceptable Health Benefits and Risks). To this end, the ARR and the NNT are useful tools for visualizing any risk or benefit. The Risk Characterization Theater has been developed to display this information in a way that will empower individuals to make their own decisions.

11. Health Effects of Smoking

Surgeon General's Warning: Smoking Causes Lung Cancer, Heart Disease, Emphysema, And May Complicate Pregnancy

Cigarette Package Warning

Issue

The subject of smoking has blackened innumerable pages since the first reports of adverse health effects appeared fifty-some years ago. Public health campaigns, scientific research, the anti-tobacco lobby, and cigarette company trials have all contributed to bring about such a change in the public conscience as would have been unimaginable half a century ago. In 1965, almost half of all American adults were cigarette smokers. By 1985, the proportion of adult smokers had fallen to about 30%.[1] In the late nineties, California introduced anti-smoking legislation, and many other places followed suit. In 2003, New York City banned smoking in bars and restaurants.[2] But according to the CDC, more than 20% of the US adult population still smokes.[3]

What exactly are the health risks that these 47 million Americans tacitly accept by continuing to smoke? This is the key question.

Background

Media reports have linked smoking with many different health effects. And as the medical studies continue, the list only grows longer. A single study is rarely "proof" that smoking causes disease X, but the body of research that now exists is extensive enough that scientists and doctors have been able to draw some pretty confident conclusions.

The 2004 US Surgeon General's Report on the Health Consequences of Smoking[4] reviewed and cited over 1,600 different sources. Taken all together, some of this evidence is so convincing that the Report infers a cause and effect relationship between smoking and certain diseases: lung cancer, oral cancer, bladder cancer, cervical cancer, coronary heart disease, stroke, chronic obstructive pulmonary disease (emphysema and chronic bronchitis), reduced female fertility, premature delivery, even cataracts, to name a few.

Other evidence is a bit weaker, merely "suggesting" a causal relationship between smoking and e.g., liver cancer or erectile dysfunction. And according to the Report, we just don't know enough to be able to claim that smoking causes decreased sperm quality or adult asthma. In these instances, the authors of this book would classify smoking as a risk factor for these conditions.

On the other hand, the Report is satisfied that certain other diseases, like breast cancer, simply aren't caused by cigarettes. Smoking even has an occasional health benefit: the Report finds that the evidence is strong for a causal relationship between active smoking and reduced risk of preeclampsia in pregnant women.

We could talk about the risk of contracting any one of the diseases associated with smoking. But some smokers will escape these afflictions, while some non-smokers will contract these diseases. In the end, how will you know whether you got heart disease because you have a family history of heart disease, because you were a lifelong smoker, or both?

What we can compare with relative ease are death rates. Everyone dies. But death rates among smokers are discernibly different than those among non-smokers of the same age, so these statistics are a way to quantify the risk of smoking in terms that are easy to understand.

Even so, absolute information about the health risks associated with smoking can be slippery and hard to interpret. The significant health end points are long-term business, so we need long-term data on real people as they live their different lives. But cigarettes have changed over the last century. So have people's smoking habits, in terms of factors like how much they smoke and what age they start. Even the people who smoke are different: men used to outnumber women greatly, but now the proportions are close to equal. And while smoking used to be common throughout American society, it is now most prevalent among the underprivileged: about a third of people below the poverty line smoke, compared to the national average of 21.5%.[1,3]

In order to make health risk data easier to interpret, researchers do their best to account for these sorts of complicating factors. Often they use statistical methods. While these studies are far from "perfect," the picture that emerges is still sobering.

Smoking Risk Characterization Theaters (RCTs)

In 1964, researchers collected information on a large number of middle-aged men living in five European countries, the US, and Japan. Twenty-five years later, they published a follow-up to their Seven Countries Study, confirming "the association of cigarette smoking with elevated risk of mortality from all causes, several cardiovascular diseases, cancer, and chronic obstructive pulmonary disease."[5]

By the end of the study, the participants were hardly youngsters any more. The risk of disease or death may or may not depend on smoking, but it definitely depends on age. So the researchers used statistical methods to attempt to account for the contributions of aging when they analyzed the results. They used similar methods to try to account for a number of other factors as well. This way, they could report "standardized" risks, which may be more meaningful especially for comparisons with different studies.

Of 2,821 men who never smoked, 1,030 died over the twenty-five year period. This is an absolute death rate of 1,030/2,821 = 0.365, or 365 deaths per thousand over the study period. The corresponding standardized death rate for this control group was 363, reported in deaths per thousand over twenty-five years.

Of the 2,465 men smoking 20-29 cigarettes per day, 1,335 died over the twenty-five year period. This is an absolute death rate of 542 deaths per thousand over the study period. The corresponding standardized death rate was 561 deaths per thousand over twenty-five years.

The absolute increase in risk for these smokers was 561 - 363 = 198 deaths per thousand over twenty-five years. The researchers were pretty confident in this result: the statistical probability of observing such an extreme difference between the two groups just by random chance would have been miniscule.

Among the participants smoking 20-29 cigarettes per day, the standardized rate of 561 deaths per thousand could be broken down as follows: 168 deaths from coronary heart disease (vs. 116 among non-smokers), 60 from lung cancer (vs. 11 among non-smokers), 28 from chronic obstructive pulmonary disease (vs. 7 among non-smokers), and 111 from other cancers (vs. 71 among non-smokers). Other heart and arterial disease, stroke, infection, accidents, and other diseases accounted for the additional 194 deaths per thousand among the smokers during the twenty-five year period.

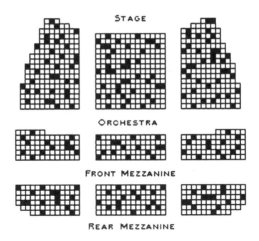

Fig. 11.1. The Seven Countries Study - the darkened seats in this theater of male smokers represent the 198 extra deaths observed over twenty-five years compared to a theater of male non-smokers. Of these 198 extra deaths, 52 were from heart disease, 49 were from lung cancer, 40 were from other kinds of cancer, 21 were from chronic obstructive pulmonary disease, and the remaining 36 were from a variety of other causes

We can use a Smoking Risk Characterization Theater (RCT) to illustrate the 198 extra deaths over twenty-five years associated with smokers in the Seven Countries Study when compared with 1,000 non-smokers (Fig. 11.1). This visual technique dramatically illustrates the health impacts associated with smoking.

Hoping to learn about the long-term effects of smoking cigarettes, other researchers collected information on the lifelong smoking habits of nearly thirty-five thousand male doctors in the UK. The British Doctors Study[6] lasted fifty years, from 1951 through 2001. The researchers observed higher death rates among smokers, in particular due to heart disease, stroke, cancer, and respiratory diseases. Longevity has been increasing rapidly for non-smokers over the past half century, but this was not true for the smokers in the study. Male cigarette smokers born between 1900 and 1930 died, on average, 10 years younger than men born in the same period who never smoked. Men who quit at age 60, 50, 40, or 30 gained back about 3, 6, 9, or 10 years of life, respectively.[6]

On the whole, lifelong smokers had a lower chance of living into old age. For example, the researchers reported the survival of those men born from 1900 to 1910 who lived from age 35 through age 80.[6] Nineteen percent of the smokers died in their forties or fifties, compared to nine percent of the non-smokers. The absolute risk reduction for non-smokers was therefore 10%. The difference in risk only got more extreme with age: 74% of the smokers died before age eighty, compared to 41% of the non-smokers, an absolute difference of 33%. We can represent these death rates in a set of Smoking RCTs. Thus Fig. 11.2 illustrates the difference in absolute death rates between smokers and non-smokers as they aged during the study. All causes of death are included.

If the conclusions of the Surgeon General's Report are not convincing enough, the results of the Seven Countries Study and the British Doctors Study clearly illustrate that smoking cigarettes is detrimental to human health. Regardless of which diseases are associated with smoking and the uncertainty in the exact number of cancers caused by cigarettes, it is clear that smoking significantly increases the risk of death at any age. Nonetheless, we each have the right to decide for ourselves the level of health risk that we find acceptable.

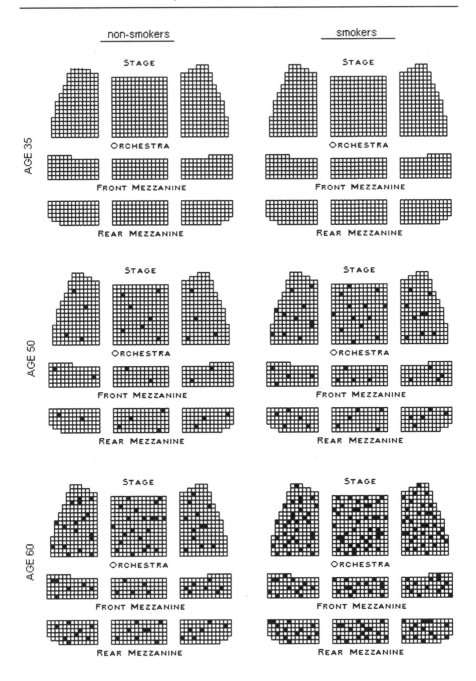

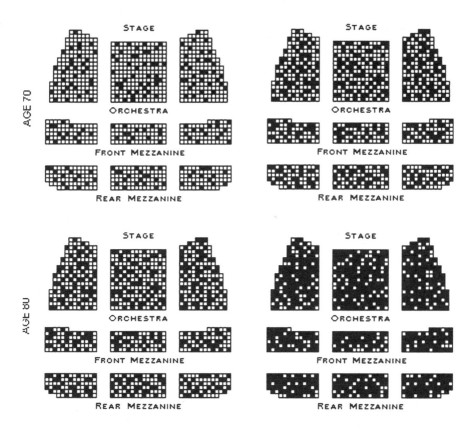

Fig. 11.2. (preceding page and this page) The British Doctors Study - these diagrams represent two groups of 1,000 male British doctors who were born 1910-1919. They were all alive at age 35, as shown in the first, all-white RCT. The darkened seats in each subsequent RCT show how many of these men died by each age milestone. RCTs on the left represent non-smokers, while those on the right represent smokers

12. Chlorination of Drinking Water and Health Risks

The United States enjoys one of the best supplies of drinking water in the world. Nevertheless, many of us who once gave little or no thought to the water that comes from our taps are now asking the question: "Is my water safe to drink?"

US Environmental Protection Agency[1]

Issue

The chlorination of drinking water has saved literally millions of lives. Adding chlorine to water kills many disease-causing microorganisms and prevents people from getting sick from the water they drink. But the benefits of destroying these pathogens come at a price. Chlorine can also attack other substances in the water, transforming them into carcinogenic disinfection by-products (DBPs). On the one hand, pathogens in unchlorinated water make people ill. On the other hand, DBPs in chlorinated water present a cancer risk. This case study examines the trade-offs.

Background

At the beginning of the 20th century, the leading cause of death in the US was infectious disease. People succumbed to such illnesses as influenza, pneumonia, tuberculosis, and gastroenteritis.[2] The young and the elderly were most vulnerable.

Early in the 1800s, people didn't really understand what caused disease or how illness could spread from a sick person to a healthy one. The pioneering work of Louis Pasteur and Robert Koch in the mid to late 1800s finally provided definitive proof that some diseases are caused by bacteria. Understanding that microorganisms were the causative agents for certain diseases was a major breakthrough.

And so this "germ theory" of disease brought about revolutionary changes in public health, engineering, and medicine. Thanks to new strategies in sanitation, vaccination, and drug intervention, the industrialized world made great strides in the fight against transmissible illness. Mortality from infectious disease plummeted from its spot at the top of the list: in 2000, the top three causes of death in the US were heart disease, cancer, and stroke. None of these diseases are infectious.

Contaminated water has always carried disease. Humans excrete many pathogens (disease-causing microorganisms) in urinary and fecal discharges. When human waste is disposed of improperly, these pathogens can contaminate surface and underground waters. If the contaminated water is used as a drinking water source, it can spread major diseases like hepatitis A, typhoid fever, amebic dysentery, giardiasis, and cholera. The afflicted suffer from diarrhea, stomach cramps, vomiting, dehydration, intestinal discomfort, and mild fever. This collection of symptoms is frequently called gastroenteritis. In the past, it was often fatal. The current death rate for such diseases in the US is fortunately quite low; it has been estimated between 0.1% and 1.0%.[3]

A classic case of public health epidemiology involving drinking water and disease occurred with an outbreak of cholera in central London in 1854. A recent article tells the story:

> Dr. John Snow sat down with a map of London, where a recent outbreak had killed more than 500 people in one dreadful 10-day period. He marked the locations of the homes of those who had died. From the marks on the map, Snow could see that the deaths had all occurred in the so-called Golden Square area. The most striking difference between this district and the rest of London was the source of its drinking water. The private water company supplying the Golden Square neighborhood was getting its water from a section of the Thames River that was known to be especially polluted. So Snow went down to Broad Street, where he suspected that one particular pump was the source of the contaminated water. And, in a gesture that still reverberates among public health scholars today, he removed the handle of the Broad Street pump. Once the pump was out of commission, the epidemic abated.[4]

Diseases from contaminated drinking water became increasingly prevalent in the burgeoning urban areas of the late 19th century. Even as the "germ theory" was gaining acceptance, cities were contaminating their own and their neighbors' water supplies with their waste. In order to reduce illness spread by drinking water, water treatment became common in US cities at the beginning of the 20th century.

The early treatment technologies were a big improvement over untreated water. Consider the example of typhoid fever in Philadelphia.[5] Between 1890 and 1906, Philadelphia's water supply was untreated, and the number of typhoid cases ranged from 200 to 680 cases per 100,000 people. Slow sand filter treatment was installed in 1906, and the number of typhoid cases fell immediately. By 1910, there were fewer than 100 cases per 100,000 people. As a further improvement, chlorine disinfection was introduced in 1913. The number of typhoid cases decreased to fewer than 20 cases per 100,000 people by 1920, and in 1935 there were fewer than ten cases per 100,000 people.

Today in the US, we take it for granted that our tap water will not make us sick. The success in controlling pathogens in US water supplies is largely the result of a hundred years of experience and the passage of regulations to establish appropriate treatment standards.

Even so, a few Americans do still get sick every year from contaminated drinking water. On average, ten incidents of disease were reported per year involving contaminated public water supplies between 1999 and 2002. For comparison, the annual average from 1976 to 1980 was 38 incidents.[6] The decrease in the incidence of disease since the mid 1980s is largely attributed to stricter regulations that focus on controlling pathogens. Most of the recent disease incidents result from mistakes, like an insufficient chlorine dose or inadequate operation of filters at the water treatment plant, or else from accidents in the distribution system, like contamination when a pipe breaks or during a flood.

Compared to other disinfectants, chlorine has the advantage of being inexpensive and effective. Even at low concentrations that aren't harmful to people, it kills many pathogens. Not only that, a little "left-over" chlorine can remain in the treated water for several days, providing continuing protection as the water flows through the city pipes on the way to residents' taps. Chlorine is effective specifically because it is very reactive and "attacks" all kinds of substances.

All natural waters contain some amount of organic matter that comes from soil and plants. This organic matter is not harmful. But when reactive chlorine is added to control pathogens, it also reacts with the natural organic matter.[7] The reaction forms DBPs. There are two main groups of DBPs, the trihalomethanes (THMs like chloroform) and the haloacetic acids (HAAs like chloroacetic acid). All these compounds share an important chemical trait: they have chlorine and/or bromine atoms caught up in their chemical structures.

Unfortunately, some of the THMs and HAAs also share another trait: several of these compounds are suspected or confirmed human carcinogens. Exposure to these DBPs may increase the risk of bladder, rectal, and/or colon cancers. Consequently, there are strict regulations in the US limiting the allowable concentrations of DBPs in treated drinking water.

In short, the use of chlorine as a drinking water disinfectant involves a tradeoff. Without chlorine, pathogens will be present, and our drinking water will make us sick much more frequently. But treating with chlorine to kill pathogens has an adverse side effect: some DBPs increase the risk of getting certain cancers. The following section presents risk characterization theaters (RCTs) to compare the likelihood of contracting an illness from untreated drinking water and the health risks of developing cancer from drinking chlorinated water.

Drinking Water Risk Characterization Theaters

Pathogenic Risk

Consider an example pathogen, the bacterium *Salmonella*. Scientists have studied *Salmonella* and other waterborne pathogens to see how exposure is related to sickness.[3] Just as you might expect, the more *Salmonella* cells you consume, the more likely you are to get sick.

Imagine a community whose water supply is contaminated with *Salmonella*. Adults drink two liters of water per day on average. If these two liters contain a total of 100 *Salmonella* cells, then 26% of the adults in the community are expected to get sick. The darkened seats in the *Salmonella* RCT (Fig. 12.1) represent the proportion of individuals who develop gastroenteritis after drinking just one day's worth of contaminated water. This is not a far-fetched example; public heath officials have measured *Salmonella* concentrations even higher than 100 cells per two liters in contaminated drinking water.

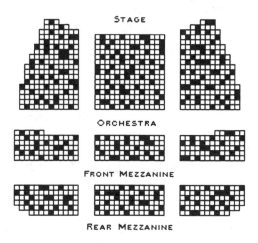

Fig. 12.1. The darkened seats represent the 260 individuals expected to get sick if the drinking water supply is contaminated for just one day. Each of the one thousand people in the theater drank the contaminated water that day and ingested 100 *Salmonella* cells

Researchers have found that if you drink the same *Salmonella*-contaminated water for an entire year, your chance of not only getting sick, but actually dying from the waterborne illness is 9.2%.[3] In other words, 92 out of 1,000 people who drink this water for a whole year are expected to die. The darkened spaces in the RCT in Fig. 12.2 represent this annual risk of death.

Ninety-two deaths from contaminated drinking water might sound like a lot, but the number shouldn't surprise us. This example considered *Salmonella*, but other pathogens could also be present in the contaminated water at the same time. Everyone has heard the travelers' mantra, "don't drink the water." Unfortunately, the people who live in areas of the world with sanitation problems don't always have that option. It is estimated that worldwide there are between 6 billion and 60 billion cases per year of gastrointestinal illness.[8,9] The World Health Organization reports that adequate sanitation and hygiene could prevent at least 90% of these cases. In short, waterborne pathogens can be major killers.

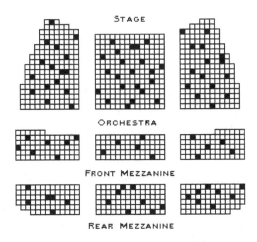

Fig. 12.2. The darkened seats in this theater represent the 92 people out of 1,000 expected to die from drinking contaminated water for a whole year. Each person drinks two liters (100 cells) of *Salmonella*-contaminated water every day

Carcinogenic Risk

The risk of getting sick from drinking water is now quite small in the US and in other industrialized countries, in large part due to the use of chlorine in drinking water treatment. However, as mentioned above, the negative side effect of chlorination is the formation of potentially toxic DBPs.

In the US, the amount of a contaminant allowed in drinking water is called the Maximum Contaminant Level (MCL). The current MCL for THMs is 80 parts per billion, and the current MCL for HAAs is 60 parts per billion.[10] These allowable concentrations correspond to a lifetime cancer risk of one in 10,000, within the EPA's acceptable risk window (as discussed in Chap. 4 and ref. 11). If we drink water that contains DBPs at the established MCL levels throughout our entire life, our risk of developing certain cancers from drinking the water is therefore one in 10,000, as represented by the RCT in Fig. 12.3.

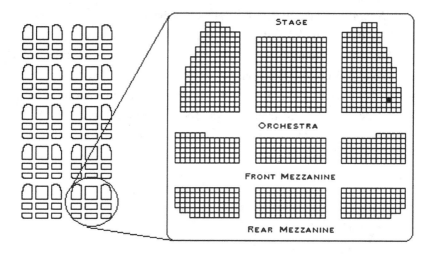

Fig. 12.3. The one darkened seat in a total of 10 RCTs represents the single person out of 10,000 who will get cancer from drinking treated water for his or her entire life, assuming that the water always contains the maximum allowable level of DBPs

The MCLs are national limits, but the concentrations of DBPs in drinking water in many places across the country are well below these levels. Information on concentrations of DBPs in local drinking water can often be found in the water quality reports that water utilities include periodically with the water bill. For drinking water with lower amounts of DBPs, the risk of developing cancer is proportionately lower. If drinking water contains one tenth of the allowable DBPs, the lifetime risk of getting cancer falls to 1 in 100,000, as represented in Fig. 12.4.

These diagrams illustrate the acute risk of getting sick from pathogen-contaminated drinking water, and they show the large risk of death from longer-term exposure to waterborne illness. Comparing Pathogen RCTs to DBP RCTs, we can see that the risk of cancer from chlorinated water is many times lower than the risk of dying from waterborne disease in unchlorinated water.

Proper treatment and chlorination remove pathogens and reduce the chance of getting sick and dying from drinking water to a very low number. At the same time, chlorination can increase the lifetime risk of cancer from DBPs up to the regulatory limit of 1 in 10,000. Consider the big picture from the *Salmonella* example: Without chlorination, no one gets cancer from DBPs, but about 92 out of 1,000 people will die every year from *Salmonella* (not to mention the deaths from all the other possible water-borne diseases). With chlorination, fewer than 1 in 10,000 will be affected by cancer from DBPs over their entire lifetime, and only about 1 out of 10,000,000 people will die from all waterborne pathogens each year. The total number of lives saved by chlorination is significant. From this point of view, the benefits of chlorinating our drinking water are clear.

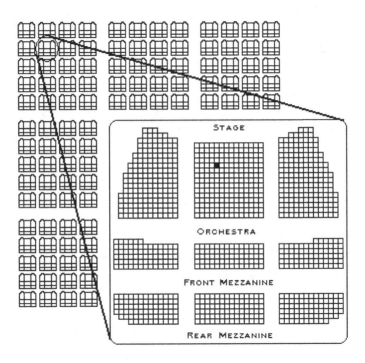

Fig. 12.4. The one darkened seat in a total of 100 RCTs represents the 1 in 100,000 risk of getting cancer from an entire lifetime of drinking treated water that contains one tenth the allowable level of DBPs

Tap Water Alternatives

Bottled water is often marketed as a better alternative to the public water supply, but it is not necessarily safer than tap water. The Food and Drug

Administration regulates bottled water, whereas the EPA sets allowable limits for contaminants in public water systems. The two agencies don't take the same approach. As a result, some bottled water is treated more than tap water, while some is treated less or not treated at all. Bottled water is much more expensive than tap water on a per gallon basis, so some water utilities even bottle a portion of the tap water that they would normally distribute through the city water pipes and sell it for greater profit. You have to read the label carefully to tell where your bottled water comes from!

Bottled water is a lifesaver during emergency situations like natural disasters. Highly-purified bottled water can also meet the special needs of people with weakened immune systems. However, fluoride is added to many public water supplies to prevent tooth decay, but fluoride is not present in most bottled water. Dentists are reporting a comeback of tooth decay, especially in young children. The increase in tooth decay is linked to drinking un-fluoridated bottled water instead of fluoridated tap water. In short, it's a good idea to consider whether the needs and benefits justify the extra cost relative to tap water.

Home water treatment units are also advertised as a better alternative to tap water. A properly-maintained home treatment unit can definitely improve water taste or provide an extra margin of safety for people who are vulnerable to getting sick from pathogens in water. But home treatment units aren't usually necessary to make water safe for healthy people. Actually, they can even lower the purity of your tap water if you fail to follow the manufacturer's instructions (such as forgetting to change the filter cartridge as often as you should). So it's important to read product information to understand what the home treatment unit actually does and how it has to be maintained.

13. Exposure to Residential Radon and the Risk of Lung Cancer

Indoor radon should be considered as a cause of lung cancer in the general population that is amenable to reduction.

Committee on Health Risks of Exposure to Radon,
National Research Council[1]

Issue

The word "radiation" often conjures up images of atomic bombs, nuclear power plants, and X-ray film. But human-made sources like these contribute only about 20% of our radiation exposure.[2] In fact, we are bombarded with radiation quite regularly, and 80% of it comes from natural sources like cosmic rays and terrestrial radiation, including radon. In the US, radon probably contributes more than half of our radiation dose.[3]

Radon is a colorless, odorless, radioactive gas that is naturally present in rocks and soil all over the world. It is formed by the radioactive decay of uranium, and it seeps out of the ground into the air we breathe. Radon gas enters buildings through cracks in foundations and walls and openings around pipes and wires. Although radon gas dissipates quickly in outside air, there is less opportunity for it to disperse inside, so radon levels can build up indoors.

The Environmental Protection Agency (EPA) and International Agency for Research on Cancer (IARC) have classified radon as a human carcinogen. There is concern that radon in homes might be causing lung cancer in the general population. Home inspectors often test for radon, and some people incur considerable expense to seal or ventilate a home with high radon levels. So a key question emerges: *what is the lung cancer risk of inhaling indoor radon?*

Background

Like other radioactive substances, radon atoms release energy as they spontaneously split themselves into smaller particles. Some of the resulting "decay products" are also radioactive, and adhere to dust particles. As they split up, both radon and its decay products emit energy in a form called alpha radiation. Fortunately, alpha radiation cannot travel far into tissue.[3] It is so weak that it cannot penetrate the dead outer layers of our skin, so radon does not pose any risk as long as it remains outside the body. However, when radon and its decay products are inhaled into the lungs, the alpha radiation can damage lung cells and disrupt DNA. DNA damage can eventually cause cancer. Since it is difficult for inhaled alpha radiation to reach cells in other organs, lung cancer is the primary cancer hazard.

Decades of research have focused on the health effects of radiation, and considerable effort has been devoted to investigating radon as a human carcinogen. The most direct way to uncover the risks from inhaling indoor radon would be to measure radon levels in homes and then observe lung cancer frequency among the people who live there. Several such epidemiological studies have been completed, but no clear answer has emerged.[1]

Direct measurement is actually harder than it sounds for a number of reasons. First, the lung cancer risk is likely to be very small at the low radon concentrations present in most homes. So a huge number of people would have to participate for a study to be able to discern a difference between people exposed to normal background radon levels and people exposed to slightly elevated home radon levels. Second, radon levels vary and people move about, so it is difficult to assess the exact amount of radon that a person has been exposed to over his lifetime. But without knowing how much radon people breathe in, how can we establish a clear relationship between radon dose and lung cancer?

Finally, smoking causes many more lung cancers than radon does. The high incidence of lung cancer from smoking makes it difficult to measure an increase in the lung cancer rate from radon exposure. To make matters worse, smoking renders your lungs more vulnerable to radon damage, and radon makes your lungs more sensitive to damage from smoking. So radon exposure increases the chance that a smoker will develop lung cancer.[1,4]

In short, estimating lung cancer risk from radon in the home based on epidemiological studies is a bit like looking for a needle in a haystack. The risk is there, but it's hard to find it.

Since it is not possible to make a valid estimate of radon-related lung cancer risk by studying people in their homes, researchers have looked elsewhere. Miners who work deep underground are exposed to higher levels of radon than you might encounter in your basement, so it is easier to study the potential health effects of radon exposure among these workers.

A National Research Council (NRC) study[1] in 1999 reviewed 11 published studies on radon-related lung cancer risk in underground miners. All in all, the studies considered about 2,700 lung cancer deaths in 68,000 men. The more radon the miners were exposed to, the greater their chances of dying of lung cancer. Based on these death rates at high radon levels in the mines, NRC scientists estimated lung cancer risk at the low radon levels we might find in our homes. Since this kind of back-estimation involves considerable uncertainty, the NRC Committee actually used several different extrapolation methods to come up with their estimates of risk for low-level radon exposure.

Combining their estimates of low-dose risk with data on radon levels in US homes, the NRC Committee figured that somewhere between 3,000 and 33,000 Americans die each year from radon-related lung cancer.[1] This broad range reflects the many uncertainties involved in the high dose to low dose estimation, as well as uncertainty about the radon levels we actually breathe in. Within the broad range, the most likely or average estimates of the lung cancer deaths from radon exposure are between 15,400 and 21,800 per year, including both smokers and non-smokers.

In 1995, about 157,400 people died of lung cancer from all causes. About 11,000 of these people were non-smokers. The NRC Committee attributed between 2,100 and 2,900 of these non-smoker deaths to radon exposure in homes.[1]

Radon Risk Characterization Theaters

Like the NRC, the EPA based its radon analysis on data from lung cancer incidence among underground miners.[5,6,7] Combining the mining data with the EPA acceptable risk level for this carcinogen, the Agency was able to develop a radon policy.

Radon concentrations are commonly measured in units of picocuries per liter of air (pCi/liter). The average radon level in indoor air is 1.3 pCi/liter, compared to 0.4 pCi/liter in outside air.[7] The EPA considers indoor radon levels over 4 pCi/liter excessive and recommends that radon controls be implemented in these homes.

At a lifetime exposure of 4 pCi/liter, the risk of radon-related lung cancer is estimated to be 7 per 1,000 for non-smokers and 62 per 1,000 for smokers. The darkened seats in the two Radon RCTs in Fig. 13.1 show these lifetime risks at the excessive indoor radon cutoff level (4 pCi/liter).

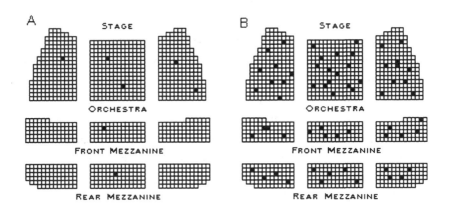

Fig. 13.1. RCTs showing the lifetime risks of developing lung cancer from exposure to radon at 4 pCi/liter, the regulatory guideline set by the EPA. The darkened seats represent the number of individuals out of 1,000 who will get lung cancer at this level of radon exposure. **A.** for non-smokers and **B.** for smokers

For contrast, the lifetime risk of developing lung cancer at the average indoor radon level is shown by the darkened seats in the two RCTs in Fig. 13.2. The lifetime risks at 1.3 pCi/liter are estimated to be 2 per 1,000 for non-smokers and 20 per 1,000 for smokers.

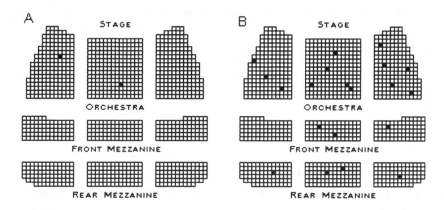

Fig. 13.2. RCTs showing the lifetime risks of developing lung cancer from exposure to radon at 1.3 pCi/liter, the average level in US homes. The darkened seats represent the number of individuals out of 1,000 who will get lung cancer at this level of radon exposure. **A.** for non-smokers and **B.** for smokers

Remember that the lung cancer risks for low-level radon exposure shown in these RCTs are estimates, calculated from data about lung cancer in miners who breathe in much higher levels of radon. From the actual radon levels in the mines to the possible differences between low and high exposure, there is a lot of uncertainty in creating these estimates. And different estimation methods yield different answers.[8] The EPA estimation method assumes that even the smallest possible radon dose presents some health risk. However, the NRC Committee[1] found that it may also be reasonable to use a different estimation method, one that assumes there isn't any health risk below a certain very small "safe" radon dose.

Nationwide Perspective

Both the EPA and the NRC Committee consider that radon is the second leading cause of lung cancer after smoking. The EPA estimates that about one out of every fifteen homes in the US is likely to have elevated radon levels.[7]

The radon level in a home is influenced by many factors including local soils and geology, house layout, construction materials and practices, and existing ventilation. High radon levels have been found in every state, and radon levels can vary from home to home, even between next-door neighbors. Professional inspectors can test for radon (price range of $75-$300) or you can purchase a do-it-yourself test kit with mail-in results ($10-$50).

The most common way to address a radon problem (over 4 pCi/liter) is to install a vent system that pulls air from beneath the house and blows it to the outside. The system is most effective if cracks and openings in the foundation and walls are sealed; the average installation cost is approximately $1,200 per home. These systems can reduce radon to a level below 2 pCi/liter, close to the average radon level in US homes. According to the current risk assessment for radon, venting in a high-radon home will lower the estimated individual lung cancer risk to values like those shown in the RCTs in Fig. 13.2 (according to EPA estimates).

The EPA estimates that 450 lives would be saved annually in the US if all of the homes with elevated radon levels were fixed to reduce the radon levels below 2 pCi/liter.[6] This is one of the reasons that the EPA recommends radon testing in all homes. The 1999 NRC Committee estimated even greater benefits: according to their analysis, eliminating radon exposures in excess of 4 pCi/liter would prevent about one third of all radon-related lung cancer deaths. But since not all lung cancers are radon-related, the total number of lung cancer deaths would only fall by 3–4%.

The risk of lung cancer from smoking is many times higher than the risk of lung cancer from inhaling indoor radon. Many of the deaths from radon exposure among smokers will not occur if the potential victims stop smoking. Therefore, the best way to reduce lung cancer deaths from radon exposure is to reduce the number of smokers.

14. Ecological Risk Assessment

It is still unclear whether ecological risk assessment will actually improve decision making and ultimately protect ecological resources.

Robert Lackey[1]

Just pick up the newspaper and you will surely find an article about environmental degradation. Human activities are responsible for massive worldwide habitat destruction resulting in the dramatic reduction or elimination of fauna and flora on every continent. Pollutants turn up at unacceptable levels in rivers, streams, lakes, soils, sediments, oceans, and groundwater systems. The effects are long-term, and in many cases they result in permanent and irreparable changes to ecosystems.

Ecological Risk Assessment (ERA) is a scientific approach used to determine the possible impacts of human activities on the environment. The EPA defines ERA as "the process that evaluates the likelihood that adverse ecological effects are occurring, or may occur, as a result of exposure to one or more stressors."[2] These stressors might be contaminants like lead, non-native species like introduced plants, habitat modifications like new housing developments, or even changes in climate. In fact, a stressor is simply a change that modifies ecological systems such as lakes, streams, forests, and watersheds. The resulting ecological risks may be limited to a local scale, such as trout disappearing from a certain stream. Or they may be regional, at the scale of e.g., the Chesapeake Bay, or even world-wide, like global warming.

Ecological Risk Assessment is in many ways parallel to human health risk assessment (which was discussed in Chaps. 4 and 5). The ecological problem needs to be defined, and the hazards need to be identified. The ecological effects need to be correlated with exposure to contaminants and/or levels of habitat destruction, and the dose-response relationships need to be determined. From all of this information, the ecological risks are estimated. Finally, risks are characterized along with major assumptions and uncertainties.

Risk managers then consider scientific conclusions from the ERA alongside policy judgments, economic ramifications, legal issues, and social concerns. They try to balance these different factors to recommend a course of action.

The description of the ecological risk assessment and management process sounds reasonable on paper. The ERA process seems analytical; it appears to be grounded in sound scientific principles. But applying these ideas in the real world isn't simple.

The difficulties begin with the very formulation of the problem: what ecological unit should we analyze? Ecosystems are webs of complex interactions between vast numbers of plants and animals. Some scientists think we should focus on a specific population of plants or animals living in the same area at the same time. Others believe it is more important to emphasize the health of a set of different organisms in varied habitats. Still others are of the opinion that we should analyze a larger ecosystem, such as the entire estuary or rain forest. There is no standard procedure for assessing overall ecological risk.

Efforts are being made to remedy this situation, but it may take decades to establish standard procedures. Even more time will be needed before the new measures can be applied to all contaminants and sites. In the meantime, there is no single, acceptable, comprehensive appraisal of risks to plants and animals.

In spite of such shortcomings, many ERA analyses have provided useful information. For example, we know that specific chemicals have negative effects in the environment. Some of this information comes from simple studies to determine the effects that occur rapidly when animals are exposed to contaminants in the wild or in the laboratory. Usually, the effect studied is death, so there is a large literature base on the levels at which particular chemicals are deadly for specific types of animals.

The story of DDT in the US is a striking example of a successful ERA. Starting in the 1940s, DDT was sprayed widely on farmland and wetlands to control insect pests that damage crops and carry disease. DDT accumulates in animal tissues, so predators at the top of the food chain can have high concentrations of DDT in their bodies. In birds, DDT interferes with eggshell formation. The shells are so thin and fragile that birds break their own eggs when they sit on their nests. Large birds of prey like ospreys and eagles are particularly affected.

The original DDT lawsuit presented scientific evidence of poor reproductive success in ospreys. It described how eggs containing high levels of DDT were not hatching. Populations of our national bird, the Bald Eagle, were also showing the effects of the use of DDT. Public awareness of the dangers of DDT increased as a result of Rachel Carson's 1962 book, *Silent Spring*. In 1972, the EPA Administrator William Ruckelshaus issued a nationwide ban on DDT.

The results of the DDT ban have been dramatic. In 1963, fewer than 500 pairs of Bald Eagles were found in the lower 48 states. By 1996, this number had increased tenfold to more than 5,000 pairs. The Bald Eagle is no longer listed as an endangered species. Ospreys have also made a comeback, increasing from fewer than 8,000 breeding pairs nationwide in 1981 to over 14,000 pairs in 1994. Equally impressive results have been observed for other birds, such as peregrine falcons and brown pelicans.[3] Unfortunately, ERA success stories like this one are the exception rather than the rule.

The primary reason for this track record is that the uncertainty in ERA is enormous. Uncertainty in human health risk assessment pales by comparison. Human health risk assessment deals with a single species, but ERA must consider many different organisms and their habitats. These plants and animals vary not only in size and life span, but also in sensitivity to particular chemicals. The uncertainty due to multiple species and population-level consequences is in addition to all the usual sources of uncertainty in risk assessment: the nature and extent of contamination, the environmental fate and transport of contaminants, the magnitude of exposure to various receptors, and the dose-response data for chemicals.

These ERA limitations cannot be overcome, but they should be disclosed. Admitting uncertainty will prevent confusion between value judgments and science. Describing scientific limitations may avoid uncertain risks being discounted. As with human health risk assessment, identifying value choices and seeking public participation can improve the quality and transparency of an ERA.

ERA aims to predict the likelihood of future adverse effects or to evaluate the likelihood that effects are caused by past exposure to stressors. Unfortunately, ERA often falls short of these goals. The following cases provide examples of the uncertainty inherent in the evaluation of ecological health. They illustrate problems that can arise in a limited situation, as well as when an issue is regional in scope.

Biological Control: Weeds and Flies

Spotted knapweed was accidentally introduced from Europe over one hundred years ago. Since then, the weed has become widespread in North America. It is an aggressive plant that quickly invades pasture, rangeland, and fallow fields. It has few natural enemies here, and livestock will only eat it when other food is unavailable.

Knapweed releases a toxin into the soil that poisons native plants. Knapweed is resistant to its own toxin, so it has an advantage over its non-knapweed neighbors. Since it crowds out more desirable species, less food is available for foraging livestock. Knapweed can even reduce crop production.[4] As a result, there are practical and economic reasons to control the spread of this plant.

Biological control agents are commonly used to deal with unwanted, invasive species like knapweed. Hundreds of predators, parasites, and pathogens have been imported and released in the US over the last century for the express purpose of trying to control exotic pests "biologically." Nowadays we try to foresee the possible problems that could arise before we introduce one species to control another. In other words, we start with an ERA.

It turns out that knapweed does have a couple of natural enemies back in its native Europe. There are two species of flies that damage knapweed buds. After extensive testing to ensure that these species wouldn't damage other plants, the European flies were introduced in Canada and Montana in the early 1970s. They are now widespread throughout much of the US and Canada.[5]

The flies are called gall flies. They lay their eggs in knapweed flower heads, where the growing larvae winter over. The plant reacts to the attack by forming lumpy "galls" around the larvae. A gall is a structure formed by abnormal growth in plant tissues. The larvae eat knapweed seeds in the flower head, and the galls take up space that otherwise would have been filled with seeds. As a result, the plant produces fewer seeds.

Although seed production has been reduced by as much as 95% in certain knapweed populations,[5] the approach appears to be insufficient. The flies make a dent, but it's not enough. The weed continues to spread, particularly in areas disturbed by human activity. Herbicides or additional biological control agents may be necessary. Time has shown that in spite of extensive testing, the predictions were wrong about the benefits of gall flies. There was just too much uncertainty. But the story continues.

Scientists recently discovered that the gall fly grubs are an attractive food source for deer mice.[6] This increases the mouse population during otherwise lean winter months. Deer mice are hosts for Hantavirus, a group of viruses that cause epidemic hemorrhagic fever and serious respiratory infections in humans. People catch Hantavirus when they come into contact with infected rodents. The prevalence of Hantavirus-positive mice is elevated in areas where there are a lot of weeds and flies. To make matters worse, deer mice are also hosts for Lyme Disease and other human illnesses.

This example demonstrates how difficult it is to determine with any degree of certainty the likelihood of adverse ecological effects from human activity. Even when the situation was thought to be confined to two specific organisms (gall fly and knapweed), things turned out to be more complicated. It is also an indication of the potential extent and magnitude of the uncertainty in most ERAs. The example used here is not intended to comment on the ecological consequences of importing natural enemies. Instead, it illustrates how potential ramifications may not be discovered until after implementing the ecological change. The example underscores the obvious: we are far from understanding the multiple, complex, ongoing interactions that make up the web of life.

Crown-Of-Thorns Starfish

Since we are avid scuba divers, my wife Elaine Rifkin and I were excited to finally have an opportunity to dive Australia's Great Barrier Reef a few years ago. Diving in this World Heritage Area was a magical experience. We entered the world of brightly colored clown fish, sea anemones, jellyfish, sponges, and corals. But the organism most essential to the survival of this magnificent ecosystem, the coral, was under attack.

The splendid corals we all recognize are actually coral skeletons. Microscopic animals (cousins to the jellyfish) inhabit the surface of the coral skeletons and are responsible for building these impressive structures. These organisms are being eaten by a voracious predator called the crown-of-thorns starfish. The dead skeleton left behind first acquires a coating of green algae. Within a couple of weeks it is encrusted with plants and animals that give it a grey appearance. Eventually, the dead coral colony collapses under the weight of all these attached organisms, destroying a portion of the reef ecosystem.

To date, starfish predation has been largely confined to the central third of the Great Barrier Reef, where the majority of tourist developments are located. The effects may have serious implications for this ecosystem, the local economy, and Australia in general.[7] Even 20 years ago, authorities acknowledged that the crown-of-thorns starfish posed a "major management problem" to areas within the Great Barrier Reef.

We know surprisingly little about the basic biology and ecology of the crown-of-thorns starfish. Over the last two decades, biologists have tried to overcome this gap in scientific knowledge. But they have to juggle a lot of uncertainty because there are many complex variables in the reef ecosystem. Given the magnitude and extent of the problem, it might not be possible to obtain useful scientific results before it's too late.

To provide data for a comprehensive ERA, researchers are studying many aspects of the starfish in its ecosystem:[7]

- dispersal and settlement of crown-of-thorns larvae
- markers to distinguish crown-of-thorns larvae from other starfish larvae
- recovery in coral and fish communities after starfish outbreaks
- predation of adult crown-of-thorns starfish

- mathematical methods for compiling data about the distribution and abundance of the starfish and its coral prey
- use of satellite photos to identify the effects of starfish outbreaks on the Great Barrier Reef
- reef sediment geological studies to see if and when starfish outbreaks occurred in the past
- studies to see if biological controls might be effective

Some of this research is currently underway, but marine biologists and ecologists acknowledge that it would take decades to conduct all these studies. Should we proceed with the decision-making process even before we have all the information we might want?

Some argue that we should not intervene until we fully understand the consequences of our actions. They fear that intervention will cause permanent and irreparable changes to our coral reef systems. Others disagree. They believe that something must be done now, that we cannot afford to wait for the scientific information. ERA doesn't have the answer. Even if we decided to "do something now," ERA doesn't tell us what to do.

To date, the largest crown-of-thorns control program was undertaken in the Ryukyu Islands, Japan. The area is a fraction the size of the infested portion of the Great Barrier Reef. Approximately 13 million starfish have been removed, at a cost of over 6 million Australian dollars (approximately 4.6 million US dollars).[7] This effort was unsuccessful in preventing further coral mortality and eradicating the starfish.

Options are limited. There is no right or wrong answer, only endless uncertainty. While research programs will continue, it is critically important to acknowledge, disclose, and emphasize this vast uncertainty and the likelihood that science may not provide a solution in the foreseeable future.

The following chapters present case studies demonstrating when ERAs can be successful in impacting decision-making, and when the uncertainty makes it virtually impossible to achieve a confident outcome. It is obviously important to understand and acknowledge early in the process the limitations imposed by uncertainty.

15. Asian Oysters in the Chesapeake Bay

The structure and dynamics of the Chesapeake Bay ecological and socio-economic systems are complex, not well understood, and subject to environmental, social, and political influences beyond the scope of management control. Consequently, decision makers are faced with uncertainty – uncertainty about the structure and dynamics of integrated physical, biological, economic, and sociocultural systems, uncertainty about how the systems will respond to the actions taken, and uncertainty about the merits of alternative outcomes.

National Research Council[1]

Estuaries are among the most complex of all ecosystems. This is where salt water from the oceans mixes with fresh water from rivers to produce one of the most unique, important, and productive of all known ecological systems. They are found on continents and islands around the world and serve as nurseries for a multitude of aquatic vertebrates and invertebrates. For millions of years these habitats have evolved to allow organisms from many phyla to develop and thrive. The dynamic nature of estuaries and the intricate relationships between flora and fauna there make this type of ecosystem one of the least understood. Scientists from many disciplines continue to study how currents, temperature, salinity, dissolved oxygen, sediment deposition, metals, and organic compounds affect the abundance and distribution of aquatic life.

Changing any of these factors will create a ripple effect throughout the estuarine system. Human-made changes which disturb the "natural order" of things generally produce a wide range of unanticipated and adverse impacts.

How can we determine the impacts that could occur as a result of the destruction of an estuarine habitat due to pollution, sedimentation, the introduction of nonnative species, or some other cause? Ecological risk assessment (ERA) is the best method, but the web of life is so intricate in estuaries that it is virtually impossible to predict, understand, and cope with many of the problems that may arise.

Unfortunately, scientists and others charged with addressing these issues often seem unable to recognize or unwilling to accept the limitations and uncertainty that are inherent in the ERA process. Such is the case in the present controversy surrounding the introduction of nonnative oysters in the Chesapeake Bay.

The Decline of Native Bay Oysters

The health of the Chesapeake Bay oyster population is of critical concern not only to the states bordering this world-famous estuary, but also to other regions in the US and the world. Why? Consider the following.

In the late 19th century:[2]

- the oyster harvest from the Chesapeake Bay was twice that of the rest of the world outside the US
- this fishery represented 39% of the US oyster harvest
- it also accounted for 17% of all US fisheries
- it employed 20% of all Americans who worked in the fishing industry
  Impressive statistics by any standard.

As recently as the 1970s, the annual average oyster harvest in the Chesapeake Bay was 15 million bushels. But in 2003 and 2004, the catch was only 53,000 bushels.[3] Many factors have been identified as contributing to this decline, including pressure from fishing, atmospheric deposition from coal burning, excessive nitrogen and phosphate due to fertilizer runoff from farms, and the addition of toxic substances to the Bay.[4] This trend has had serious economic ramifications for everyone involved with the oyster industry. The decimation of Chesapeake oysters has also contributed to the overall decline in the biological diversity and ecological health of this magnificent estuary, because oysters are efficient filter feeders that remove contaminants from this aquatic ecosystem.

While it is generally agreed that these factors have contributed to the rapid drop-off in the oyster population, the decline of this industry is most directly attributed to the presence of two microscopic disease-causing organisms: MSX and Dermo.[1]

The Microscopic Culprits: MSX and Dermo

MSX was first discovered in nearby Delaware Bay and then, in the late 1950s, spread to oysters in the lower Chesapeake Bay.[5] The name MSX stands for "multinucleated sphere unknown" and was used before this single-celled organism was classified; it is now called *Haplosporidium nelsoni*. The disease Dermo is also caused by a single-celled parasite with the scientific name *Perkinsus marinus*. Dermo had been found in Chesapeake Bay oysters around 1950, but it wasn't until the 1980s that it started to cause serious problems to oyster populations.[6]

During the 1950s, it became evident that the presence of these microscopic organisms could have long-term, irreversible consequences for the oyster industry in the Chesapeake and Delaware Bays. It also became very clear that little was known about these pathogens. Federal and state government agencies and academic institutions began to conduct research on the distribution, life cycle, transmission, infection rates, reproduction, host response, and resistance of MSX and Dermo. In addition, programs were set up to investigate environmental parameters (salinity and temperature), oyster mortality rates, histology, and pathogenicity associated with these diseases. While research costs are difficult to estimate, by the end of the 20th century, considerable expenses had been incurred trying to find ways to understand and stop the spread of MSX and Dermo.

About forty years ago I (author Rifkin) became part of this research effort when I went to work at the Rutgers University marine lab in Bivalve, New Jersey. The nearby town called Shellpile consisted of a number of oyster shucking houses. The oyster boats would leave from Bivalve and return to Shellpile with oysters dredged from the bottom of Delaware Bay.

There, the oysters were shucked and sized, packed in cans, put on ice, and shipped throughout the US.

Using a modified oyster boat, we scientists also went out and dredged for oysters, not for the pleasure of eating them, but for MSX research. Dredging involves dragging a heavy, basket-like contraption along the bottom of the Bay, scraping up oysters and anything else in its path. It was hard work, particularly in the winter when the temperature dipped below 20 degrees Fahrenheit and the wind exceeded 25 mph. When the dredge was hauled up, all fish and invertebrates inadvertently captured by the dredge were thrown back in so that these organisms could once again be part of this environment. The live oysters were collected and brought back to the lab for study. In the lab, the oysters were shucked, "fixed" or preserved in alcohol or formaldehyde, cut into thin sections, stained, and prepared for viewing under a microscope.

Microscopic examination told us which oysters were infected with MSX, the level of infection, the intensity of the infection, and the effect on gills, reproductive organs, and other parts of the oyster. These data could then be used to determine how, when, and where the disease was spreading in Delaware Bay. Analogous research efforts were being conducted in the Chesapeake Bay and in research labs up and down the East Coast of the US. Similar but more sophisticated research programs are still asking many of the same questions almost half a century later.

Native Chesapeake Bay oysters, *Crassostrea virginica*, are very susceptible to MSX and Dermo, particularly in waters with high salinity – which accentuates the problem, since oysters tend to grow more rapidly in saltier waters. Attempts were made to plant young oysters in waters with low salinity and then transplant them when they were more robust and could better withstand the infections caused by these diseases. These efforts did not achieve the desired results, due in part to less-than-optimum conditions in waters which were less saline and to the presence of predators like the oyster drill, a snail which bores a hole through the oyster's shell to eat its flesh.[7]

Starting in the 1960s, after the initial epidemic outbreaks of the diseases, selective breeding programs designed to produce resistance in *C. virginica* were initiated at Rutgers University and at the Virginia Institute of Marine

Science. These breeding programs used survivors from infected populations to produce more resistant offspring.[8]

Ultimately, this approach failed to work. Something new and dramatic would have to be tried to revive the Bay's oyster population.

The situation was becoming grave, so ominous in fact that it led to serious discussions about the possibility of introducing a foreign species of oyster into the Bay, one which would be more resistant to MSX and Dermo.

The Debate about Introducing Foreign Oysters

Non-indigenous species have either intentionally or unintentionally been introduced to estuaries and other ecosystems throughout the world.[9] In fact, oysters have been intentionally transported more than any other marine species.[10] Yet, to date, it has been impossible to predict whether a species will turn out to be "invasive," becoming overly abundant and spreading from the site of introduction.

Making predictions is especially daunting in complicated ecosystems such as estuaries. Since estuaries are typically used for fishing, shipping, and recreation, they generally contain a relatively high number of non-native species. Though most scientists agree that only a small percent of introduced species will ultimately become invasive, there are plenty of examples where this has occurred – with devastating consequences. Just look at the millions of dollars spent annually to combat the nonnative zebra mussels that encrust water intake pipes in the Great Lakes region.[1]

According to a recently prepared comprehensive report by the National Research Council (NRC),* "It is extremely difficult to predict whether a marine species has the potential to become an 'invasive' or a 'nuisance' species."[1] Generally speaking, it seems that the more degraded and the less biologically diverse an estuary is, the more vulnerable it is to invasion. Case studies in different regions throughout the world indicate that benefits and disadvantages associated with the introduction of exotic species appear to depend on site-specific conditions. What happens in one situation has little or no predictive value for another situation.[1]

After a preliminary evaluation of the ecological risks which could result from the introduction of a foreign oyster to the Chesapeake Bay, the Asian or Suminoe oyster (*Crassostrea ariakensis*) was selected as the oyster which had the best chance of "supplementing" the stock of native oysters.[1] Shortly thereafter, Maryland proposed legislation advocating the introduction of this nonnative oyster to the Chesapeake Bay. This proposal has generated considerable debate.

Those advocating the introduction of *C. ariakensis* to the Bay – the Governor's Office, the Maryland Department of Natural Resources, and the commercial seafood industry – point to evidence that this species may be resistant to MSX and Dermo. They argue that we need to act quickly in order to give the watermen a crop to harvest and provide a mechanism to filter out contaminants.

Those opposed raise legitimate concerns regarding the overall negative effect that this decision could have on this aquatic ecosystem. Environmental groups, sport fishermen, natural resource officials in Delaware and New Jersey, and the National Academy of Sciences (NAS) support a bill which would delay introducing Asian oysters to the Bay. They argue that additional study is essential in order to answer questions regarding the potential adverse environmental impacts that could result from the introduction of a foreign species of oyster to the Bay.

Both sides seem to agree that scientific research will, *in a reasonable time frame*, provide enough information to make a sound decision on *C. ariakensis*. But history tells us otherwise. ERA simply has not evolved to the point where it can be used to effectively assess risks in complex ecosystems.

The Limitations of Scientific Research

When I was conducting research on MSX many years ago, there were unanswered questions as basic as these: How is MSX transmitted? Does this pathogen have intermediate hosts? How many life stages are in its life cycle? How did it get to the Chesapeake Bay? Over forty years later, we still don't have the answers we need for assessing the risk.

All of this earlier research was focused on the impacts on native oysters (*C. virginica*). Now, ecological risk assessments would need to be expanded to include impacts from the introduced species as well. That expansion exponentially raises the level of uncertainty. It is unlikely that new scientific evidence would be able to make a significant contribution in the near future in the face of so many unknowns. Nonetheless, major players requested that the NRC conduct a study on the matter.

The Chesapeake Bay Foundation, an environmental group formed to protect the Bay, sent the NAS a letter which stated, in part, the need

...for an independent technical study [...] to describe the state of our knowledge of *C. ariakensis*, identify key gaps for which research would be required, and assess the risks inherent in utilizing this species to support Chesapeake Bay fisheries. (Letter from William C. Baker, President, Chesapeake Bay Foundation to Ms. Morgan Gopnik, Director, Ocean Studies Board, National Research Council; January 9, 2002.)

A letter from the EPA, Region III, stated a concern "... over the lack of scientific knowledge which would be necessary for any agency to make an informed decision" on the proposal to introduce the Suminoe oyster to the Chesapeake, and underlined

...the dire need for guidance in identifying research that would be essential to support an informed decision, and our interest in obtaining an independent evaluation of research results, risk assessment needs, and oyster management options.... (Letter from Diana Esher, Acting Director, EPA, to Dr. Bruce Alberts, President, NAS; January 9, 2002.)

A letter from Barbara Mikulski (US Senator from Maryland) to the EPA and NOAA stated that

...recent research suggests that a non-native species, *Crassostrea ariakensis*, may grow faster and survive disease better than the native oyster. Supporters of saving the Bay, including the oyster industry, the watermen, and environmental organizations, agree that we need further information about the potential benefits and impacts of introducing this species to the Bay. (Letter to the Honorable Christie Whitman, Administrator, EPA, and Vice Admiral Conrad C. Lautenbacher, Jr., Under Secretary and Administrator, NOAA; January 22, 2002)

And finally, a letter from the Chesapeake Bay Commission says,

Introducing a non-native species is not a decision to be taken lightly. An independent technical study is needed to describe the state of our knowledge, identify research priorities, and assess the risks inherent in utilizing this species to support Chesapeake Bay fisheries. (Letter from Ann Periri Swanson, Executive Director, Chesapeake Bay Commission, to Ms. Morgan Gopnik, Director, Ocean Studies Board, National Research Council; January 16, 2002.)

The NRC formed a Committee on Nonnative Oysters in the Chesapeake Bay and proceeded to conduct a comprehensive study. The final report, *Nonnative Oysters in the Chesapeake Bay*, was released in 2004.[1] It analyzed and assessed three options: 1) prohibiting the introduction of nonnative oysters to the Chesapeake Bay; 2) the introduction of open-water aquaculture of sterile Suminoe oysters; and 3) the introduction of reproductive Suminoe oysters.

Not surprisingly, the NRC committee concluded that the level of uncertainty made it virtually impossible to characterize the ecological risks of maintaining the status quo (option 1) or introducing sterile or reproductive *C. ariakensis* (options 2 and 3). Regarding option 3, the NRC concluded that "large gaps in biological knowledge exist for both native and non-native oysters, and the biology of both species needed to be understood in the broader context of long-term environmental change in the Chesapeake Bay." Some of the critical gaps in knowledge presented in the NRC report are listed in Box 15.1.[1]

The NRC also recommended some "longer-term research goals" which include: the development of a model of oyster larval dispersion in the Chesapeake Bay; an experimental design for a breeding program which would result in disease tolerant native oysters; and the determination of "the genetic and physiological bases for disease tolerance or resistance of native oysters."

Realistically, it would take decades to develop a research plan, conduct the research, and interpret the findings for *any* of the identified critical knowledge gaps. Obtaining the needed information and integrating it into a strategic plan is, at this time, difficult to imagine. As of 2006, unanswered questions regarding the life cycle and transmission of the MSX and Dermo parasites and basic questions concerning oyster resistance still exist. Therefore it seems highly unlikely that findings from additional research on *C. ariakensis* will be forthcoming in a meaningful time frame.

Box 15.1. Critical gaps or areas of uncertainty regarding the introduction of non-native oysters in the Chesapeake Bay (adapted from ref. 1).

- Develop methods which will result in the detection and elimination of introduced pathogens
- Determine the susceptibility of the Suminoe oyster to another pathogen (*Bonamia ostreae*) which has been linked to *C. ariakensis* mortality elsewhere
- Develop a better understanding of *C. ariakensis* biology in the Chesapeake Bay, particularly its growth rate, life cycle, larval behavior, and larval settlement patterns in different hydrodynamic regimes; size-specific post-settlement mortality rates; and susceptibility to native parasites, pathogens, and predators incorporating salinity and temperature dependencies
- Obtain, assess, and evaluate data on the likelihood that sterile Suminoe oysters will become fertile
- Evaluate the range of conditions (e.g., water flow) which will result in fertilization
- Determine the ecological interactions of *C. ariakensis* and *C. virginica* at the juvenile, adult, and gamete life stages
- Determine the genetic diversity of different geographic populations of *C. ariakensis* and other related Asian species of the genus *Crassostrea* and the extent to which they might respond differently to the Chesapeake Bay environment

---

Without this information, decision-makers will not be able to count on science to help them determine whether or not to introduce the Suminoe oyster to the Chesapeake Bay. While great strides have been made in assessing ecological systems, great care needs to be taken not to overestimate our ability to understand and predict the impacts associated with the introduction of organisms to aquatic ecosystems.

In light of this situation, the words of the Nobel Laureate economist Dr. Friedrich Hayek are worth noting:

There are definite limits to what we can expect science to achieve. This means that to entrust the science – or to deliberate control according to scientific principles – more than the scientific method can achieve may have deplorable effects. This insight will be especially resisted by all who have hoped that our increasing power of prediction and control, generally regarded as the characteristic result of scientific advance, applied to the process of society, would soon enable us to mold it entirely to our liking.[11]

While many environmental problems can be resolved by focused and directed research over the short term, this is not one of them. Individuals and organizations responsible for preparing environmental impact statements, conducting ERAs, and dealing with scientific aspects of this issue should acknowledge the limitations in the practical application of their research. Since public monies are generally used to fund this research, funding agencies should demand a higher level of accountability.

It's time to reframe the debate – to acknowledge that we can't rely on science to resolve the current oyster crisis in the Chesapeake Bay. There simply isn't enough time. Those responsible for making the difficult choice of whether to introduce Asian oysters or to maintain the status quo should recognize that any decision will be replete with uncertainty and risk. Regardless of the outcome, early recognition of the limitations of science will result in a process better able to reach a risk management decision in a timely and efficient manner. ERAs need to become far more sophisticated before tackling an issue of this scope and magnitude.

Perhaps those institutions requesting the NRC study simply wanted verification that additional study should be required before a decision could be made. But whatever their motives, the scientists associated with these prestigious institutions were surely not surprised by the NRC study results. As one author observed, "When harm will be substantially irreversible, as in the case of carcinogenic exposures, extinction of species, or acid-rain contamination of lakes and forests, the problem of how long regulators should wait for 'enough' information to enable reliable scientific judgments is likely to be controversial."[12]

Given the enormity of this oyster industry problem and the obvious inability of science to identify the best solution with any degree of certainty, decision-makers at the highest level will have to depend on sound advice, good judgment, and a sense of how much risk can be tolerated. For the time being, our government leaders and members of the scientific community need to get comfortable with uncertainty in situations like this. This is certainly a wiser approach than pretending that scientific research will be a panacea.

*The National Research Council was organized by the National Academy of Sciences (NAS) in 1916. The Council has become the principal operating agency of the NAS and the National Academy of Engineering (NAE) in providing services to the government, the public, and the scientific and engineering communities. The NAS and NAE are private, nonprofit societies of distinguished scholars engaged in scientific and engineering research. The Academies have a mandate that requires them to advise the federal government on scientific and technical matters.

16. Chromium and Sediment Toxicity

*Therefore, barring any contradictory data, this information provides suffi-
cient justification to remove chromium as an impairing substance in the
Inner Harbor.*

Maryland Department of the Environment[1]

Baltimore's Inner Harbor is an historic seaport, the number one tourist at-
traction in the city, and an iconic landmark. It is a branch of the Patapsco
River, which begins about fifty miles inland and terminates as a large tidal
inlet of the Chesapeake Bay. Over the past few decades, the Harbor has
been transformed from an industrial waterfront into one of the best examples of urban renewal in the country.

Where oil refineries and storage tanks once stood along the banks of the
Patapsco, upscale condominiums with spectacular water views now line the
Harbor's edge. Factories that spewed out metals and organic pollutants
have been replaced with chic retail stores and expensive restaurants. The
river merges with the Chesapeake Bay, so yachts moored in the Inner Harbor
have easy access to the recreational amenities of that world-class estuary.
Indeed, the dramatic conversion of the Inner Harbor into Baltimore's jewel
is one of the main reasons a prominent travel guide listed Baltimore as one
of the ten most desirable tourist destinations in the US.

Unfortunately, the contamination in the Patapsco River did not disappear along with the industrial sources of that pollution. The sediment lying
beneath the Harbor's waters is a case in point. In spite of efforts to clean
up the area, recent studies show that Harbor sediments are toxic to bottom-
dwelling organisms.[2] Scientists agree that sediments are responsible for
adverse effects on the flora and fauna of the Patapsco River, but there is
intense debate as to the cause of this toxicity. This uncertainty underscores

the inherent limitations of ecological risk assessment (ERA) in effectively addressing environmental problems in complex aquatic ecosystems.

Government Agencies and Water Quality

The passage of the Federal Clean Water Act (CWA) established regulations to protect, maintain, and restore the environmental quality of the nation's waters. The CWA first defines the use of a particular body of water (e.g., fishing, swimming, public water supply) and then applies appropriate limits on pollutants to ensure that this defined use is not compromised. However, laws and strict standards for pollution control don't translate readily into action. The CWA was first passed in 1972 and has been updated since, but reversing the degradation of the nation's rivers, streams, and lakes is proceeding at a glacial pace.

In accordance with a specific section of the CWA, Maryland and other states are required to develop a list of lakes, rivers, streams, estuaries, and other water bodies that have been impaired by contaminants or excess nutrients. As the state agency primarily responsible for ensuring that contaminants in Maryland waters do not exceed established water quality criteria, the Maryland Department of the Environment (MDE) develops such a list every other year and sends it to the EPA for approval. The Baltimore Harbor is on that list.

The EPA listing includes not only the impaired water body but also the "impairing substances," or contaminants. An impairing substance is included if it exceeds established water quality criteria or other such limits. These criteria, which are usually developed by the EPA, are set to ensure that there will be no toxicity to sensitive aquatic organisms or humans. Water quality criteria relate to levels of pollutants or contaminants that are dissolved in the water and bioavailable, i.e., readily able to enter the tissues of fish or other aquatic organisms.

Baltimore Harbor sediments contain high levels of three metals: lead, zinc, and chromium. MDE tentatively determined that these three metals should be listed as impairing substances. As a result, action would be required to reduce the amounts of these pollutants. The decision was presented to interested parties at a public meeting. These stakeholders included representatives from federal and state regulatory agencies, the environmental community, industry, academia, and the general public. All were anxious to hear what MDE was going to do about the environmental contamination in the Baltimore Harbor, which was responsible for adverse impacts on aquatic organisms and significant damage to natural resources.

The environmental community viewed MDE's findings as the beginning of a long-awaited cleanup of the Harbor. They hoped those responsible for toxicity in the Harbor were finally going to be held accountable for past and present abuses. After all, the river had been a virtual dumping ground for industrial wastes and nutrients from agricultural facilities. The environmentalists were cautiously optimistic that, this time, something was actually going to be done to solve the problem.

Others didn't share these sentiments. MDE's decision and any future proposed action was of particular concern to one company that was tied to chromium discharges. MDE's decision to list chromium could result in significant costs.

The final decision about whether or not chromium qualified as an impairing substance in this case would be the responsibility of the EPA.

Historically, industry tends to ask for more scientific evidence that the pollutants they are generating are truly responsible for adverse impacts to the ecosystem. The environmental community tends to take the opposite position: even if the underlying science is uncertain, go ahead and do a cleanup so that conditions will replicate those found in pristine waters. For their part, federal and state regulatory agencies move slowly and deliberately when it comes to imposing sanctions on companies that are providing jobs and tax revenues. Finding a solution agreeable to all can prove to be very difficult.

Could Ecological Risk Assessment Work in this Case?

The company needed to make sure that MDE's decision was based on sound science. So it brought in some experts to discuss the chromium issue and provide advice on how to proceed. The company's consultants prepared a summary of the facts and a suggested a course of action. Here are the highlights of what they presented:

- There was ample scientific evidence that sediments in the Baltimore Harbor were toxic to aquatic organisms. Therefore, MDE had good reason to be concerned about this situation.

- The consultants cautioned, however, that there didn't appear to be any conclusive evidence regarding the specific causative agent(s) responsible for this toxicity. Therefore, implicating chromium, zinc, or lead was not warranted at that time without further analysis.

- Published data indicated that the three metals of concern were found in the water column at concentrations well below the EPA's and Maryland's water quality criteria.

- The decision to list chromium as an impairing substance was therefore based on chromium concentrations in the Harbor *sediments*, not on concentrations in the water. While the EPA had developed specific criteria for contaminants in the water column, acceptable chromium levels in the Harbor sediments would be based instead on sediment "guidelines." Guidelines are not the same as criteria.

- The science used to develop guidelines is not as rigorous as that for criteria, so the level of uncertainty associated with guidelines is considerably higher. There are always caveats regarding the use of guidelines for regulatory purposes. As a result, guidelines are not usually used as enforceable standards. But neither the EPA nor MDE had sediment criteria for these three metals; only guidelines were available.

- The consultants also advised the company to look at the peer-reviewed scientific literature and evaluate the results of previous ERAs. They said that while ERAs were not particularly useful when looking at potential impacts to complex ecosystems, these assessments could often be used for a specific contaminant such as chromium.

- Finally, the experts advised their client to focus on the scientific evidence which correlated toxicity with levels of chromium in sediment. They explained that if toxicity to aquatic organisms went up when levels of chromium in the sediment was elevated, the company would probably have to bite the bullet and accept MDE's decision. On the other hand, if it could be demonstrated that there was no relationship between chromium levels in the sediment and toxicity, that would be reason to dispute MDE's findings and conclusions. Fortunately, they would be able to conduct this analysis, since there were a number of peer-reviewed articles that contained information on toxicity and levels of chromium in different areas of the Baltimore Harbor.

MDE's decision to use sediment guidelines had raised some fundamental questions and concerns regarding the appropriateness of their approach. MDE recognized the scientific and technical difficulties involved. And MDE knew that the fundamental uncertainty regarding the use of guidelines for regulatory purposes was bound to generate considerable controversy, so they actively sought public comment on their tentative decision.

Taking a Closer Look at Chromium

Contaminated sediments can be found in fresh and marine ecosystems throughout the world. In many instances, they have been associated with ecological and potential human health risks.[3] Some classes of contaminants are considered problematic in sediments, including some metals and certain organics.[4] Numerous metals fall into this category, such as lead, arsenic, chromium, mercury, and cadmium. The organic contaminants of concern are those that are not soluble and have a strong tendency to absorb or stick to sediment particles. These include many pesticides and other chlorinated compounds.

Quantifying the toxicity due to metals in sediments is especially challenging because a metal's form significantly affects its mobility, bioavailability, and toxicity. The form of a metal is determined in turn by geological conditions and the chemistry of the water-sediment system.

Since practically all contaminated sediments contain mixtures of organics and metals, it is virtually impossible to single out which agents are responsible for ecological risks. In certain instances, scientists can shorten the list of possible culprits by eliminating some chemicals, but even then the specific causes of sediment toxicity generally cannot be confirmed.

To make this situation even murkier, sediment quality guidelines are usually based on total concentrations of a pollutant, thereby ignoring how different forms of the chemical can differ in bioavailability, toxicity, and mobility in the environment. Such was the case for chromium.

MDE was receptive to all perspectives on this issue, so a few months after the stakeholder meeting, MDE scientists listened to the company's analysis. The analysis was limited to the toxicity of a single contaminant in one specific location, so it was appropriate to apply the principles of ERA.

The company made a formal presentation to MDE, explaining that in aquatic systems chromium exists primarily in two distinct forms: a trivalent form identified as Cr(III), and a hexavalent form, Cr(VI).[5] These two forms have markedly different toxicity and behavior. To all intents and purposes, Cr(III) is not toxic at environmentally relevant concentrations. Cr(VI), on the other hand, is a known human carcinogen and is toxic to aquatic flora and fauna at relatively low concentrations. Given these facts, lumping both forms of chromium together as "total chromium," as in the sediment guidelines, is not scientifically acceptable when the objective is to predict toxicity.[6] Apparently, at the time the guidelines were developed, no one gave any thought to determining the levels of the different forms of chromium.

The company presented results from peer-reviewed journals to support the view that using sediment quality guidelines based on total chromium was inappropriate and not scientifically justifiable. Using data from field studies, they demonstrated that there was no correlation between toxicity to aquatic organisms and concentrations of total chromium in Baltimore Harbor sediments. Given the absence of this relationship, it would be very difficult to support a decision to list chromium as an impairing substance.

Furthermore, there was strong evidence that the chromium in sediments in Baltimore Harbor, as well as in most sediments throughout the world, is predominantly if not entirely Cr(III). Environmental conditions in sediments tend to favor the formation of Cr(III). The company didn't dispute the contention that the Harbor sediments were toxic, but rather challenged the assumption that chromium was causing the toxicity.

Since industry consultants' conclusions tend to be viewed as biased and suspect, confirming evidence from well-respected EPA scientists proved to be a valuable part of the presentation. Recent EPA publications in peer-reviewed journals were used to buttress the company's scientific arguments. These EPA studies dealt with the complex relationship between geochemistry, chromium speciation, and toxicity to small, shrimp-like, bottom-dwelling marine invertebrates called amphipods. Experiments demonstrated three main findings: sediment with Cr(III) is essentially not toxic to amphipods; Cr(III) is rarely found in the dissolved or bioavailable form; and Cr(III) is generally attached to organic particles and cannot pass through cell membranes readily.[7,8]

In contrast, research has demonstrated that Cr(VI) is soluble. Once it is taken in by an animal, Cr(VI) can penetrate cell membranes. After undergoing modifications, it can interact with DNA and other substances within the animal's cells.[9] There is clear evidence that exposure to certain levels of Cr(VI) can result in significant human health and ecological risks. Cr(VI) is a potent human carcinogen when exposure is by inhalation. Dermal contact can result in allergic contact dermatitis, and ingestion can result in a number of adverse systemic effects.[10] Similarly, the bioavailability and toxicity of chromium to aquatic organisms has been associated with dissolved Cr(VI).[11] Toxicity from exposure to chromium in different media – air, water, sediments – is also generally associated with Cr(VI).

Furthermore, the EPA scientists determined that if substances called Acid Volatile Sulfides (AVS) were found in sediments, it would mean that the Cr(VI) would be converted (or "reduced") to the non-toxic Cr(III) form. Their experiments explored the relationship between the presence of Cr(VI) and AVS. They found that AVS forms only under conditions where there is no oxygen. As it turns out, Baltimore Harbor sediments are anoxic (i.e., without oxygen), just like most other sediments underlying lakes, rivers, and estuaries. Studies of freshwater sediments conducted by the US Geological Survey showed similar evidence of Cr(VI) reduction to Cr(III) in the presence of AVS.[12] The findings of these studies strongly suggest that the presence of AVS in sediments produces a natural process that serves to eliminate Cr(VI).

Responding to the Skeptics' Concerns

Although the evidence presented by the company was very compelling, the environmental community was still concerned. They reminded MDE that chromium, due to its widespread industrial use in the United States, has been introduced to the environment (water, soil, sediment, or air) as a byproduct or waste material of many processes: manufacturing steel and other alloys; preserving wood; tanning leather; and electroplating metals. Chromium has also been a component in refractory bricks used in high temperature furnaces, in pigments and dyes, in drilling muds, in rust and corrosion inhibitors, in textiles, and in toner for photocopiers.[10] Since chromium is so versatile, it's not surprising that chromium contamination is widespread; the US EPA's National Priority List database lists 135 sites around the country with chromium-polluted sediments.

There were still unanswered questions, too. Even if additional sampling and analysis demonstrated that sediments were predominantly Cr(III), how could we be sure it wouldn't convert to toxic Cr(VI) if conditions changed in the future? What about the ecological impacts on aquatic organisms ingesting chromium-contaminated sediments? And, if everyone could agree that it would be better to not have any form of chromium in the Harbor, why not remove it just in case? MDE acknowledged that these issues needed to be addressed.

Even though MDE had spent the better part of a decade developing an approach using sediment quality guidelines, they acknowledged that the company's arguments were persuasive. Therefore, they concluded that additional data should be collected before they made their determination if chromium was or wasn't an impairing substance responsible for toxicity in the Baltimore Harbor. MDE decided to resample Harbor sediments.

This time, the sampling emphasis would not be on total chromium in sediments. Instead, it would focus on determining levels of dissolved, bioavailable chromium, zinc, and lead in the Harbor water column. Scientists would also sample water in the spaces between sediment particles, known as porewater. If the levels of Cr(VI) found in the water column and in the porewater were higher than the water quality criterion, MDE would assume that Cr(VI) was responsible for toxicity, and appropriate remedies would be implemented. If, on the other hand, levels of dissolved Cr(VI) were clearly below the criterion, chromium would be taken off the list of substances impairing water quality in the Baltimore Harbor and its tributaries. After discussions with the EPA, MDE also decided to measure concentrations of AVS.

MDE developed the experimental design for their sampling and analysis plan in conjunction with the University of Maryland. Samples were collected, bottled, and sent to an independent laboratory for analysis. The results were presented at the next stakeholder meeting. Since MDE's findings were not released prior to the meeting, everyone was on edge waiting for the scientific verdict.

The results were conclusive. Concentrations of Cr(VI) in the water column and porewater were at least an order of magnitude (ten times) lower than the EPA's established water quality criteria. Essentially all of the chromium found in the sediment was the non-toxic Cr(III). Finally, every sample confirmed the presence of AVS, further supporting the contention that there was no Cr(VI) present in these sediments.

In its report to the EPA, MDE stated:

This report provides an analysis of the data used to determine the Inner Harbor […] impairment listings. It also includes recently collected data that indicates that although sediment toxicity is present in the Inner Harbor […], the source of the toxicity cannot be attributed to Cr. […] However, the segments will remain listed as impaired for biological community impacts due to sediment toxicity.

Barring the receipt of contradictory data, this report will be used to support the removal of total Cr as an impairing substance in the Inner Harbor.[1]

While the company saw this as very good news, MDE didn't forget the questions and concerns raised by environmentalists. The report's Executive Summary also states:

Although the waters of the Inner Harbor […] do not currently display signs of toxicity due to Cr, the State reserves the right to reassess the impact(s) of all Cr species on the environment due to future changes in Baltimore Harbor water quality, including, but not limited to the improvement of dissolved oxygen levels due to a reduction in nutrients. Furthermore, the State reserves the right to require additional pollutant controls in the Inner Harbor […] if evidence suggests that

Cr from either basin is contributing to water quality problems within Baltimore Harbor.[1]

Interestingly enough, even the company agreed that further assessment of possible adverse impacts to the environment due to chromium-contaminated sediments was a good idea. In fact, they provided funding to a Center at Johns Hopkins University (JHU) to attempt to answer some of the questions posed by MDE. The agreement was that JHU researchers would evaluate the likelihood that chromium would remain in the trivalent form if conditions were to change in the upcoming years. The company agreed to fund this work even though JHU insisted that the research be conducted independently and that the findings could be published in peer-reviewed journals, regardless of the results. While this type of arrangement is not the first of its kind, it is certainly unusual.

A Less-Uncertain Future for the Harbor

This case study demonstrates how and when ERAs can be effectively used to determine whether an environmental stressor (like a contaminant) is responsible for an impact (like toxicity). This ERA worked because it focused on one single contaminant – chromium – at one specific site – the Baltimore Harbor. It made use of results from scientific literature, but it also relied on an analysis of recent, site-specific data to reach a conclusion regarding the toxicity of chromium-contaminated sediments. By distinguishing between forms of chromium, it also illustrated how site-specific assessments of chemical mobility, bioavailability, and toxicity are important when evaluating whether individual chemicals have a detrimental effect on the environment.

Uncertainty was minimized by the ability to define the issue clearly and to obtain relatively straight-forward results. The regulatory agency (MDE) could base its risk management decision on sound science. With an approach like this one, ERA can be a very useful tool.

An understanding of "the science" doesn't always drive the regulatory process. It did in this case, but only because several of the major players were open-minded. MDE was willing to accept scientifically valid research and findings that contradicted their previous views and positions. The EPA also showed open-mindedness when it agreed with MDE's science-based findings. And the company's decision to fund a truly independent study – which might reach conclusions that could have an adverse financial impact on the company – was laudable.

Part III

Perspectives

17. The Physician's and Patient's Perspective

by Bob Sheff, MD, Guest Author

How do I Get the Best out of the Health Care System?

In order to get the best health care possible, you need to learn how to be your own *patient advocate*. One critical part of being a wise patient advocate is to build a *partnership* with your doctor. One of the key skills in building that partnership is being able to *communicate* with your doctor on medical issues. You need to develop a common language with your doctor so you can honestly and candidly discuss his recommendations to you. The day is long gone when the doctor-patient relationship was based on the doctor telling the patient what the diagnosis was and what the treatment plan was, and the patient accepting everything without question.

The good news is that modern medicine is based on a high degree of respect for patient autonomy. That is also the bad news, because wisely exercising that autonomy means you, the patient, have to be informed and thoughtful. How do you become an informed patient? Certainly a large part of this is based on what your doctor tells you. An open and trusting partnership with your doctor is critical for the type of honest communication that allows a patient to have all his questions answered. In addition to what the doctor tells you, as a patient you also have independent sources of medical information.

Whether we like it or not, today both physicians and patients are inundated with scientific information. In order to practice medicine at its best, the physician needs to keep up with these latest research findings. Likewise the patient is reading and hearing a steady flow of medical research findings and recommendations. Newspapers, TV, and radio quickly pick up possible medical breakthroughs and publicize them to the nation and the world. How do you possibly know which are significant to you and which aren't? As your own patient advocate you want to develop the necessary skills to be able to analyze the vast array of medical information you are exposed to and understand clearly the conclusions and recommendations being offered. In order to communicate well with your doctor, you need to have an understanding of the significance of what your doctor is recommending. *This book will give you tools to understand what you read, see in the media, and hear from your doctor.* It will enable you to improve your communication and therefore your partnership with your doctor.

A Medical Focus!

While this book deals with both environmental and medical health risk characterization, this chapter will focus on just the medical health risk aspects. I will do this from the perspective of both the trained physician and the experienced patient, as I have been both. The key to communicating well with your doctor is rooted in the skills of patient advocacy. I have learned them over the years, and I have learned how to teach them.

I began my career as a practicing physician. Over a period of years I became involved in the leadership of my large multi-specialty medical group, eventually serving as its Medical Director and President. I also played roles for BlueCross BlueShield of Maryland, serving as a Medical Director, Senior Vice-President, and President of their four HMOs. I have also had my own experiences as a patient confronting life-threatening diagnoses. From these experiences I learned how critical it is for a patient to be his own medical advocate. In my book, *The Medical Mentor – Get the Health Care You Deserve in Today's Medical System*, I teach people how to accomplish this. One aspect of being your own medical advocate is how you deal with medical information and how you communicate with your doctor. These are skills that are very relevant to the lessons of this book, *The Illusion of Certainty. This chapter will teach you, the physician or patient advocate, an approach to maximizing the lessons of this book.*

How will this Impact My Relationship with My Doctor?

In order to get the most from your medical care, I believe you need to establish a true partnership with your doctor. This partnership is based on mutual respect and a willingness to discuss honestly any topic related to your medical care. On the one hand, you want your doctor to be able to give you his best advice on the course your treatment should follow. On the other hand you want to be comfortable in asking the doctor questions about his recommendations. You also want to be able to explore alternative approaches. Some of these alternatives might even mean a different doctor treating you.

I believe *medicine is an art*, not a pure science. By this I mean that although there are strong scientific underpinnings to the many decisions you make as a patient, there are also subjective and value components that I call the art of medicine.

In order to get the best care from your doctor, you need to be able to discuss the scientific basis and the subjective basis of her recommendations. The scientific basis is the extensive medical research that has been accomplished and is still ongoing. If you don't have the ability to discuss the results of studies on which your doctor is basing her recommendations, it is very hard to be an informed partner. This does not mean you have to understand all the science involved. It does mean that when an article provides numbers for the risk or benefit of something, you need to be able to *understand what the numbers are saying*. That understanding will allow you to be a true partner with your doctor. It will enable you to discuss how you feel about the proposed intervention. It is not that you want to debate an article with your doctor. It's that you want to have a common language to discuss how your medical options align with your personal values and wishes. You need to be on the same page as your doctor if you are going to discuss what treatments are compatible with your own sense of the risk you are willing to take. *These lessons will improve your communication with your doctor, and they will let you form a closer partnership with him.*

How do I Know Who and What to Believe?

Being a successful physician or patient advocate means understanding the validity of what you hear or read. One aspect of this relates to the source itself. This means noticing who the author is. If it is a journal, is it peer reviewed? If it is a web site, is it unbiased? Another aspect of validity relates to understanding whether the way the data are analyzed and presented allows you to make decisions related to your health care. This area is where *this book can be invaluable to you.*

You want to be clear how confident you are in the recommendations being made. The recommendations are based on the conclusions the researchers drew from their data. As a patient or a physician you want the researchers to make it clear what criteria they used to reach those conclusions. Researchers formulate medical recommendations when they convert the scientific data produced in their study into a proposed action plan for the patient. This inherently involves some judgment on the part of the researchers. How they present the data can change your impression of the importance. Let's look at some of these factors and how they impact you.

Should I Care about the Difference Between Cause and Effect vs. Risk Factors vs. Association?

The authors of this book do the patient and the physician a real service by emphasizing the distinction between cause and effect vs. risk factors. I will not attempt to repeat their thorough discussion. It may be helpful, however, if I relate some of the discussions I had with the authors after reviewing a draft of Chap. 2, "Cause and Effect vs. Risk Factors." The reason for relating our discussions to you, the reader, is to highlight how thoughtful you have to be in this area.

The authors were discussing a woman considering mammography. They correctly said that a lump cannot be considered a *cause* of breast cancer. However, they then defined a lump as a *risk factor*. To a physician, this was not the correct terminology. They define a risk factor as a "condition…that has an association with but has not been proven to cause…a disease." That is a good definition of a risk factor, but is broader than I have found usually used in clinical practice. *This illustrates that professionals in different disciplines can use different terms for the same thing.*

In medicine, a lump is felt to be a sign of a disease. When a patient comes to a physician with her own observations about her health, we call what the patient observes a *symptom*. What the physician observes or finds on examining the patient we call a *sign*. A risk factor, a symptom, and a sign of a disease all have one thing in common: there is an *association* or correlation between them and the disease. This means that they tend to occur in a patient with that disease at a greater frequency than predicted by chance.

The strength of the association (how often they occur in patients with a given disease) guides physicians in assessing the significance of symptoms, signs, and risk factors. Signs and symptoms are most often seen in medicine as results of the disease. They alert us to look for other evidence that the patient already has the disease. Risk factors alert us to the possibility that the patient has or may develop a disease. They challenge us to be more alert for evidence of that disease in the patient.

The importance of this story to the patient advocate is that it highlights how careful you have to be when discussing medical conditions. You want to use that same sensitivity when discussing medical research. Finding associations between things is a critical goal of research. We use words and numbers to express those relationships. As an educated physician or a prudent patient advocate, you want to be very careful about how these relationships are described.

Another lesson for the patient advocate in evaluating Chap. 2 is about the *selection of what research is reviewed.* The authors worked diligently to find an article about mammography that had a database in it they could evaluate. The book is teaching you to evaluate data. So it was important that the study they cite provide data to examine. The authors are careful to alert the reader that they feel the area is controversial. Many physicians might disagree both with the conclusion of the article and with the statement that the use of mammography is controversial. This disagreement is important to you as a patient advocate.

On almost every topic in medicine you can examine the literature and find conflicting recommendations. What are you to do as a patient? I believe the wise patient advocate will take information she hears and discuss it with her physician. This is part of the communication and partnership you want to have with your physician.

As you gain analytic skills from this book, don't be lulled into thinking it's all in the numbers. As the authors carefully point out, there are significant subjective elements that are not in the numbers. These subjective elements cause some of the *uncertainties* in medical research. Your job as a patient is to analyze the information presented as carefully as you can and then discuss your conclusions and concerns with your physician. The skills learned in this book should facilitate that process.

Why is Using Absolute Risk So Important?

How do we know if we should follow the recommendations from a given study? The answer is that you need to be confident that the risk/benefit information in the study is accurately portrayed in a manner that is meaningful to you in your decision-making. You need to know, not just think, that the results are meaningful to you. Helping patients and physicians to make that distinction is what this book is all about.

As the authors of this book will show you, using *relative risk and relative risk reduction* can be very misleading. This should be surprising because we are bombarded with relative risk statements. As the authors continue their discussion in Chap. 2, you learn why *absolute risk and absolute risk reduction* are much better tools for analyzing risk relationships.

When you use the relative risk approach the results often appear more significant than when you use the absolute risk approach. This is especially true when the absolute risk is very small. Why is this? As the authors explain, this is because if the risk being analyzed is very small, then doubling it for instance might still be a very small risk in absolute terms. However in relative terms, doubling something is a 100% change.

If you are an author invested in the importance of your findings, your results often appear more significant if you use relative terms. But if you are a patient trying to determine the significance of a risk being described, you will have a much clearer picture of the findings if they are in absolute terms.

What is the physician or patient to do? First, see if the data are complete enough in the article to convert the results to absolute terms. As you will learn in this book, if the data are there, the conversion is generally not too difficult. If the data are not there, take your article and your questions to your physician. Scientific articles normally have contact information listed. Either you or your doctor can contact the researcher and ask for the data necessary to do an analysis in absolute terms. An additional strategy is to look for further articles on this same topic. *You want to avoid settling for the relative analysis. If you base your decision on such incomplete data, you could be doing yourself a real disservice.* As a wise patient advocate, you want to put in the effort to find the best information.

What is the Risk Characterization Theater (RCT)?

At this point you may well be thinking that this is a lot of heavy duty statistics. As you read this book, I believe you will come to realize that on the contrary, this is an approach that converts numbers into concepts. The creation of the *Risk Characterization Theater (RCT)* by the authors is a real service to both physicians and patients. The RCT is a visual way for you to assess risk and benefit numbers. If you just read or hear risk assessment numbers, it is often difficult to appreciate what they are telling you. The RCT converts the impact of the risk into an easily understood picture. It is a device that patients and physicians can utilize to assess risk data from any source. As you review the authors' examples, notice how helpful the RCT is. I suggest you become familiar enough with the RCT that you could construct one on your own. As you will see later in this chapter, the RCT is a tool we call on to guide us better in our medical decision making.

Does the RCT make the Decision for Me?

The good and bad news is, "No!" The RCT is a way of visualizing statistical results. Then you need to take these results and decide along with your physician on what you want to do. The case study in Chap. 6, "Vioxx™ and Heart Attacks," is an excellent example. As the authors show you in the Vioxx™ RCT, if 1,000 people take Vioxx™, there will be 16 more people who experience cardiovascular events than if they did not take Vioxx™. That does not tell you what to do. Rather it is a tool for you to assess the risk. You then need to discuss this with your doctor and decide what treatment options you have. Are there alternative safer treatments that are as effective? Is this a risk you are unwilling to take no matter what the benefit? Are you so bothered by your condition that this is a risk you are willing to take? As you can see, *the RCT lets you better appreciate the risk* or benefit of a medical intervention. Whether you are willing to take that risk or enjoy that benefit is up to you.

What are Some of the Pitfalls to Reading Medical Recommendations?

As you have read about in this chapter and will learn in depth in the book, there are clearly pitfalls for the unprepared patient trying to read medical literature. That is why you hear me so consistently saying that the wise medical advocate takes his thoughts and questions on medical research and discusses them with his physician.

I had some very interesting conversations with the authors in preparing this book. They deserve all the credit for the concepts in this book, and for the presentation. I was invited to write this chapter late in the process, after they had the basic framework in place. Let me share with you some of the issues we discussed as I reviewed their individual chapters.

One thing to keep in mind is the *role of screening*. When we talk about a routine screening test, we are talking about a test recommended to patients at average risk. If you have a relevant family history or some other factor that puts you at high risk, then it would not be considered routine screening. What will be apparent to the reader is that in some cases, there is more consensus among physicians about what we recommend to our patients than the literature can support. It can be debated whether that is good or bad, as I will discuss later.

What do I do if I Have Concerns about the Conclusions of an Article?

As you will hear frequently in this chapter, the primary thing a patient can do is take the article and his concerns and discuss them with his physician. If you wish to clarify your thoughts first, one alternative is to review more research about the same issue. The article òn Mammography in Chap. 2 discussed above is a good example. The authors used an article by Gotzsche and Olsen published in 2000.[1] As I note above, many physicians disagree with the conclusions and recommendations in this article. If you want to explore this area further, you might choose to also review an article by Tabar et al. published in 2003.[2] This article also has a satisfactory data set for the reader to analyze. As a physician or patient advocate, you want to do more than just read their conclusions. You want to review and compare their data sets. Particularly you want to make sure you are looking at data as *absolute risk (AR)* and *absolute risk reduction (ARR)*. Let us do such a comparison between the Gotzsche and Olsen article and the Tabar et al. article.

The data for the Gotzsche article is provided for you in Chap. 2 and I have used those figures in absolute terms for this comparison. In the Tabar article, they report raw mortality data. This allowed me to calculate the comparison numbers in absolute terms. One very important step when doing this type of comparison is to *be sure you are reviewing data over the same length of time*. In this case, I have converted both numbers to annual AR and ARR. This was necessary as the Gotzsche study was over a 12 year period and the Tabar study was over a 20 year period. So what do we find?

The annual AR of the control group according to Gotzsche is 0.4 in 1,000, for the screening group it is 0.3 in 1,000, and therefore the ARR is 0.1 in 1,000 annually. For the Tabar data the annual AR of the control group is 0.5 in 1,000, for the screening group is 0.25 in 1,000 and therefore the ARR is 0.25 in 1,000 annually.

Thus far, I know these are a lot of numbers. Let's convert these numbers into a visual presentation that is easier to relate to. We will take the authors' tool, the *Risk Characterization Theater (RCT)*, and compare the ARRs.

As you learn in detail in Chap. 3, "Reframing the Debate," the RCT is a way of analyzing data using your visual skills. If you do this you would have two sets of ten theaters each, side by side (10,000 seats in each set). In Gotzsche's theaters you would have 1 out of the 10,000 seats darkened. In Tabar's you would have 2.5 out of the 10,000 seats darkened.

The darkened seats represent the actual annual additional risk of death due to breast cancer which is avoided by mammography screening according to each researcher's data. You have to decide how different these RCTs are. As you visualize these two theaters, a question to ask yourself is, "is one substantially different to me than the other?" Gotzsche looks at his data and in his paper states that screening mammography is "unjustified." Tabar looks at his data and states in his paper that "mammography screening is contributing to substantial reductions in breast cancer mortality." The annual difference is one and a half seats in ten theaters of 1,000 women. What would *you* conclude from these two studies individually and together?

This example shows us *important lessons about reviewing research, especially in cases where we are concerned about the conclusions.* First we see how if you want to evaluate data, you have to convert the information into a form that you can understand. Second, when comparing studies, you have to be careful that the study periods are the same, or you need to correct for this. Third, different authors can reach very different conclusions with very similar data. *The most important lesson in this book is that you have to make your own decision about what is important to you.* The tools in this book will help you to visualize risk and benefit issues better. But the decision is up to you. Your doctor can help and guide you, but you have the final word. Hopefully the lessons you will learn in this book will help you make those decisions.

Why do these Absolute Risks and Absolute Risk Reductions Seem So Small, When I Know that Breast Cancer is One of the Major Cancer Risks?

This question highlights one of the major challenges to physician and patient alike when looking for guidance in the medical literature. One aspect of the confusion is related to the issue we discussed earlier, *the length of the study*. Because these studies covered different lengths of time, we converted the results to *annual risk*. This technique is helpful as it allows direct comparison between the studies.

The problem is that the patient is usually concerned about *lifetime risk*, not just the risk in a single year. It is tempting to try to extend the annual average over a larger number of years. In this example one might say that the maximum period of breast cancer risk begins at age 40. If we assume a woman will live to be 85, then we might want to take the annual ARR from each study and multiply it by 45 years to calculate the lifetime risk. However, this approach makes a number of significant assumptions of questionable validity.

As you will find discussed by the authors, physicians and patients need to be aware of *uncertainty* when they are evaluating any research. By attempting to take short term studies and extrapolate them over a lifetime, we are introducing more uncertainty into the process.

If we can't estimate long-term effects from short-term studies, where can we find meaningful information? One approach is to look at published lifetime risk data to create a framework for evaluating the significance of medical risks. *Lifetime risk data* can be found in various places. The websites of the National Cancer Institute and the National Institutes of Health are excellent sources for cancer data.[3] The most recent data from these sites state that the lifetime risk of death from breast cancer for a woman is 2.9%. That means that the RCT for the absolute lifetime risk of breast cancer death would have 29 out of the 1,000 seats filled.

It would be ideal for physicians and patients if there were research studies that calculated ARR in terms of lifetime risk. Unfortunately, that is not how medical research works. The reader, therefore, has to stay vigilant to the impact of the length of a study on the results and conclusions published. When you talk to your doctor about a study, be sure to ask about this important issue.

Are there Other "Uncertainty" Factors that Decrease Benefits in the Study Groups for Screening Studies?

Yes there are, and the patient advocate wants to be aware of them. For instance, the populations examined in screening studies are usually different than the general population. By definition, screening is considered for the population of patients who are at average risk. *High-risk patients* are usually evaluated more thoroughly than the screening population. This means that some patients who will get the disease are not in the study.

In addition, most screening tests have false positive and false negative results which tend to make them less efficient in selecting people who may come down with a disease. Patients with *signs or symptoms* of the disease are not considered screening patients. Another issue is that screening protocols are usually designed for patients in a certain age group. *Patients younger or older than the screening group* will not be considered in the study.

A final factor is the *aggressiveness* of the disease an individual patient has. If a patient gets e.g., a very aggressive case of breast cancer, even diagnosis in a screening study may not affect the patient's survival. Not surprisingly, the sum of all these factors is often a significant difference between the lifetime risk you might predict from a given study, and the actual lifetime risk of that disease when the lifetime cause of death statistics are reviewed.

How is Lifetime Risk Helpful in My Healthcare Planning?

As we have been discussing, lifetime risk information can be of great help in letting you focus on those diseases that are of the greatest danger to you. For instance, the lifetime risk of death from heart disease is 280 out of 1,000. In comparison the lifetime risk of death from colorectal cancer is 23 out of 1,000. If you think about what the RCTs would look like, you can appreciate how effective this tool is. The heart disease theater would have about one quarter of the seats darkened (280 seats), while the colorectal cancer theater would have about 2% (23 seats) darkened. These RCTs let you assess your personal risk from each condition. They make it easy for you to conclude which disease is the greatest risk to you.

I want to be clear on the message this information can give you. If unfortunately you develop an uncommon disease, it is still a potentially devastating event for you. Rare diseases can be just as dangerous as common ones. Therefore, progress in diagnosing and treating any disease is valuable. However, if you are healthy and planning your strategy for where you want to put your efforts in disease prevention, then statistically, trying to avoid common diseases would be expected to be more beneficial than trying to avoid uncommon diseases. This is where the lifetime risk tables can help physicians and patients in planning a health care program.

An example might help. If you are a man, your lifetime risk of dying from prostate cancer is about 2.9%. Your lifetime risk of dying from thyroid cancer is 0.04%. Let us look at RCTs to better visualize these numbers. In the usual 1,000 seat theater, you would have 29 seats darkened in the prostate cancer theater and less than half of a seat darkened in the thyroid cancer theater. Clearly the greater risk to you is prostate cancer. Obviously, this doesn't give you permission to engage in risky behaviors that would increase your chance of developing thyroid cancer. Rather, this use of lifetime risk data and the RCTs lets us see that you would want to put your efforts into preventing prostate cancer.

Is Relative Risk Data of any Help?

Relative risk data can be helpful, but not when viewed in a vacuum. As the authors demonstrate, relative risk numbers can be very misleading. This is because RR numbers can show a very dramatic change which may not be important to the reader. What do I mean by this? What I mean is that if you have a very, very small chance of developing a disease, and then cut that in half, you have a 50% RRR. How important is it to you if a risk which was already one in one million, is now one in two million? It is probably not very important! Don't misunderstand me; any risk reduction may be helpful. However, where do you want to put your energy and emphasis?

So what is a possible role for relative risk analysis? I believe physicians and patients can *use RR and RRR as a means to screen study results*. If the RR and RRR are low, the study is not likely to be helpful to you in planning your health care. If it is high, than you need to decide how significant the study is. As the authors discuss in detail, converting to absolute risk (AR) and absolute risk reduction (ARR) is the optimum strategy. Alternatively you could use the lifetime risk table to assess whether the probability of developing that condition warrants further effort on your part. Again let me stress the importance of discussing any such considerations with your physician!

How Clear are the Recommendations for Colorectal Cancer Screening?

Colorectal cancer screening is a great example to discuss. There are four different screening protocols which are recommended by the relevant medical associations. There are also variations among these recommendations. The main four options for screening are Fecal Occult Blood (FOB), sigmoidoscopy, combined FOB and sigmoidoscopy, and colonoscopy.

There are multiple studies evaluating the impact on mortality of the independent use of FOB screening and sigmoidoscopy screening. Both of these techniques decrease the mortality from colorectal cancer. The recommendation to use combined FOB and sigmoidoscopy has not been evaluated in a large controlled study. However, medical logic suggests you would get more benefit from combining these two screening methods than from either alone.

Although there is no accepted large study documenting the efficacy of colonoscopy as a screening tool, there are several medical reasons to believe that colonoscopy should be the most effective treatment option. Therefore, it is included as an option in most screening recommendations. In fact, the American College of Gastroenterology considers colonoscopy every 10 years as the "preferred" method of screening. The disadvantage to colonoscopy is that it has more significant complications than the other screening tests. These complications have been well-documented, and the risk numbers for them are available. As your own patient advocate, you want to discuss the pros and cons of these screening options with your doctor. Now in addition to the colorectal cancer screening options discussed above, let me focus on the studies used as the example in Chap. 10, "Colorectal Cancer Screening."

The authors summarized the results of three screening studies using FOB and follow-up diagnostic colonoscopy if FOB was positive. These studies, which demonstrated a death benefit of approximately 1 in a thousand, represent a very robust data set for colorectal cancer screening.

First we should note that the authors reported that researchers recommend FOB screening should be done at least every two years. As you may notice in the chapter, two of the three studies were European studies. In the American literature, the accepted standard is to use FOB screening every year. The importance to the patient advocate is to remember that *we now live in an international medical community*. When you are reviewing studies, you need to be aware of where they are performed. It is not that the American recommendation is right and the European is wrong. It is rather that, as we discussed earlier, *medicine is an art* and there is a subjective component to evaluating research.

As we discussed above, the *length of the study* is one critical element to consider when you evaluate a study. The three studies in Chap. 10 are combined to report absolute risk numbers. They followed patients for over a period of up to 13 years. When the researchers conclude that without screening the colorectal cancer mortality rate was 2.9 per 1,000, that risk is for the patients followed over the length of the study. As your own patient advocate, you are concerned about the remainder of your life, not some shorter interval. For example, since most colorectal cancer screening recommendations begin at age 50, you want to know the risk from that age to the end of your life. The shorter time of a study can alter the risk *analysis*.

The *nature of a screening population* is something else you have to be aware of when you are reviewing research. By definition you are only screening people at average risk. That means they do not include any high risk individuals or anyone who has any signs or symptoms of the disease. The importance to you in evaluating studies is that the incidence of a disease in a screening population will be lower than in the general population.

The colonoscopy discussion gives us an excellent example of how these multiple factors come into play. Colorectal cancer is the second most common cause of cancer death in the United States (lung cancer is the first). The latest numbers from the National Cancer Institute show that the *lifetime risk of colorectal cancer is 23 per 1,000*. The physician and the patient advocate need to keep this in mind as they evaluate individual studies. As you can see from the studies from Chap. 10 discussed above, a given study can only tell you so much. You have to take that information and relate it to the larger medical picture to decide how useful it is as a guide for decision-making.

Should We Screen for Prostate Cancer?

Physicians and patients will find that the authors highlight some very interesting issues in Chap. 7, "Prostate Cancer Screening." Physicians have been screening for prostate cancer for decades by doing a digital rectal examination (DRE). However, now there is also a screening blood test, the Prostate Specific Antigen (PSA). The PSA is more sensitive than the DRE. This test was developed as a means of searching for evidence of recurrence or spread of prostate cancer in patients who had already been treated for this disease. When the potential for using this test as a screening test became apparent, it rapidly became widely utilized.

The problem the authors note is that there does not appear to be a major paper which documents that PSA screening improves patient survival. Simply put, we don't know whether cancer screening will help men live longer! This makes it impossible for the authors to calculate an absolute risk reduction and draw a risk characterization theater.

This prompted some interesting discussions with the authors. We do know that PSA screening will find more men with prostate cancer than DRE alone. It would seem that if we found more cancers, we could save more lives. However, this has not yet been proven. This may be because the PSA test was so quickly adapted by practicing physicians that the definitive study was never done. Does this mean the test isn't helpful and should not be performed? Not necessarily. It is possible that the definitive study will find that people who undergo PSA screening live longer than those that don't. We just don't know. Again we do know that many knowledgeable physicians in the field believe that this test will provide early detection of prostate cancer.

However, even if screening finds more cancer, that doesn't mean it will necessarily save more lives. The problem is that a man may have prostate cancer without it ever being a problem for him. In autopsies of men who died of other causes, one third of men under 80 had prostate cancer and two thirds of men over 80 had prostate cancer. Since we know many men die of aggressive prostate cancer, these autopsy findings tell us that *there are at least two categories of prostate cancer*. There are the aggressive cancers that according to the National Cancer Institute account for the death of approximately 29 out of every 1,000 men. There must also be non-aggressive cancers which are not a threat to the health of those who have them.

Thus the challenge physician and patient face is how to decide whether you have an aggressive prostate cancer that needs to be treated, or a non-aggressive one that will not impact your life expectancy or life satisfaction. There is active research on multiple fronts to attempt to answer that question. Again, many knowledgeable physicians in this field believe that they can advise patients as to who should pursue treatment and who should not.

What is the wise patient advocate to do? Is it foolish to have a test before its ultimate impact is proven? I do not believe there is a simple answer to this question. This is where your partnership with your physician is so critical. I think you need to discuss the multiple issues regarding the risks and benefits of PSA screening and of treating any suspected or proven prostate cancer with your physician. Current recommendations in this area are being based largely on scientific logic and small series and anecdotal evidence, but not on the type of large definitive study we would prefer. It doesn't mean the recommendations are wrong. It does mean *you want to understand the uncertainty behind the current recommendations*. You also want to understand the risks and benefits of acting or not acting.

What are the Lessons in the Cholesterol and Statins Chapters?

Chapter 8, "Elevated Cholesterol: A Primary Risk Factor for Heart Disease?" and Chap. 9, "Statins, Cholesterol, and Coronary Heart Disease," reveal some fascinating issues for doctors and patients to consider. Let us consider the lessons from the authors' RCTs for elevated cholesterol. It's important to note that the RCTs are based on additional *annual* deaths. When a patient speaks with his physician about his own risk from elevated cholesterol, I believe he wants to be thinking about his *lifetime* risk. As we discussed earlier, the lifetime risk of death from heart disease is 28%. This is 280 seats in our RCT of 1,000 seats. This is another example of the importance in considering the *length of a study* when analyzing it.

We see the same issue when we look at the RCTs for the impact of statin therapy. In these studies, if you did not have a history of cardiovascular disease (CVD) then your benefit from taking statins was about 3%, and your RCT had 30 darkened seats out of 1,000. However, the authors tell us these studies were over approximately a five-year period. Likewise the benefit for those who already had a history of CVD was calculated to be about 7% over five years.

We can again see in Chap. 8 how data analysis is unfortunately less straightforward than it appears. However, it does highlight the care we must take in analyzing research papers. There are many other factors to consider when deciding if particular research is relevant to your care. These articles show how the RCT is an excellent tool for understanding the data. But you need to think about the data before you use the RCT, and this is a skill you want to develop. It is one of the questions you want to ask your doctor when you bring her questions about research you have encountered.

Why do You think that the Pharmaceutical Companies Advertise the Drop in the Cholesterol Number?

This is an interesting question because it raises the issue of the *outcome* of a study. Using the statins as an example, why do you take them? Is it to lower your cholesterol reading, or is it to extend your life and avoid cardiac disease? The latter, of course! You only care about the cholesterol number because you think it is a measure of cardiac risk. As discussed by the authors, this may not be as true as it first seemed.

If you are a patient or a physician, it is important that the measured outcome of the study be the outcome you are truly interested in. That is why *mortality* studies are so helpful. If the study you are reviewing shows a significant drop in absolute mortality, this is very helpful to you in assessing its significance. The problem with pharmaceutical companies advertising the effect of statins on cholesterol levels is that they are touting the wrong outcome! You want to be aware of this issue whenever you see research results.

Does the RCT Overstate Data?

I don't believe the RCT understates or overstates data. What it does is convert data into a visual pattern. By doing so it can, I believe, dramatize the data. Chapter 11, "Health Effects of Smoking," demonstrates this point. We all know there is plenty of evidence that smoking is bad for your health. This is easy to appreciate when you see the RCT for the Seven Countries Study, which demonstrates the additional 198 deaths per 1,000 over 25 years. This RCT shows the absolute risk reduction (ARR) for non-smokers.

As you review the multiple RCTs′ prepared from the British Doctors Study, you see how the RCT can also be used to show absolute risk (AR). I believe it creates a striking visual lesson as you compare the non-smokers to the smokers at each age level. Note how easily you can convert between AR and ARR: you need only subtract the AR for the non-smokers from the AR for the smokers to produce a series of RCTs showing the excess deaths (ARR) at each age level. This is why I believe the RCT is such an excellent tool for physician and patient to better understand research data.

Why isn't Lung Cancer Screening Discussed by the Authors?

Lung cancer kills more Americans than any other cancer. In fact, lung cancer kills more people than the combined totals of colorectal cancer, breast cancer, and prostate cancer. If you look into the history of screening for lung cancer you find how the "right answer" changes over time. There was a long period of time when chest x-rays were obtained as part of a routine physical examination. This was because it was well-documented that you could find lung cancers on chest x-rays. However, subsequent excellent studies demonstrated that patient survival was not being improved. In other words, by the time you found the lung cancer, it was too late to treat it. Therefore routine chest x-rays for lung cancer screening were no longer recommended.

The good news is that research is ongoing. Promising studies are evaluating low-dose CT scanning of the chest. Early partial results suggest that this method may help to diagnose lung cancer early enough to obtain a cure. As of yet, no studies are available to fill out an RCT. However, I would encourage both physicians and patients to be on the lookout for them. When such studies are published, apply the lessons learned in this book to assess the significance of the data.

As you follow the ongoing research in lung cancer screening, note that these studies are a little unusual. Instead of focusing on people who are at average risk, like most screening studies do, the researchers are screening only high-risk individuals. The target group is people with significant exposure to smoking or to second hand smoke. It is a good example of how careful you have to be in evaluating research. You want to be sure you are clear on how terms are being utilized – in this case, the word "screening."

Is there a Secret Revealed in this Book?

Is there a secret in this book? Yes! The secret is that in understanding scientific data, you have to be comfortable with how the data are presented. If the information is not presented in a way that is helpful to you, you need to convert it into a helpful format. That is why you need to learn how to use absolute risk and absolute risk reduction. It is also why you may find it very helpful to create your own Risk Characterization Theaters (RCTs) when reviewing an article. You need to view the data in a way that helps you make decisions wisely.

Is there a secret to reading this book? Again, yes! The secret is that this book is all about the process of reviewing data. The authors have selected articles with adequate data sets for proper analysis. They have tried to find representative articles in each of the topical chapters. Sometimes different researchers analyze data and come to different conclusions on the same subject. In other words, these are controversial issues, and researchers have differences of opinion. This, in turn, results in different recommendations for medical intervention. I feel it is important for the reader to focus on the data and the process rather than on the recommendations. Learning the process of proper and easy data analysis is the question at hand! If you are interested in the recommendations, use the tools the authors teach you in this book in your evaluation. Then, as any wise patient advocate would, discuss your analysis with your physician.

Remember, *the wise patient advocate knows not to analyze medical information in a vacuum.* You want to be able to examine the data and see if the risk or benefit described seems important to you. If it does and if you feel it is relevant to your medical care, then take that information to your doctor and ask his opinion of its relevance.

The best medical care is founded on a healthy *partnership* between patient and physician. The patient is comfortable taking any question to his doctor. The doctor considers all the patient's questions seriously and answers them to the best of his ability. The skills cultivated in this book should be a step forward in allowing that partnership to thrive.

18. Acceptable Health Benefits and Risks

The Concept of Acceptable Risk

Previous chapters of this book emphasize empowering individuals to participate in discussions about the significance and importance of medical benefits and environmental health risks. Those chapters stress the value of having the appropriate data in a format (e.g., Risk Characterization Theaters, absolute benefits and risks instead of relative benefits and risks) conducive to meaningful involvement. This book encourages the reader to determine his or her level of acceptable risk before making a decision regarding the benefits of screening tests and drugs or the risks from environmental contamination.

But how do we determine our level of acceptable risk? How did the EPA settle on what should be the level of acceptable risk for exposure to cancer causing substances? How does the medical community determine what are the acceptable benefits and risks associated with screening tests and drugs?

In determining an acceptable level of any risk, how we perceive the risk is a key factor. Perceptions, in turn, are based on values, views, opinions, feelings, and beliefs. As individuals, we make decisions regarding acceptable risk every day. Should I learn how to SCUBA dive? Is flying safe after 9/11? How often should I wash my hands? How much money should I put in stocks, bonds, CDs, or money market funds? Based on knowledge and experience, we use our judgment to make these choices – choices that require us to define our own level of acceptable risk.

When you judge how acceptable a risk is, you weigh a number of factors. Is the risk voluntary (e.g., SCUBA diving) or involuntary (e.g., air pollution)? How serious is it? Are you sure? Would any unfortunate effects be permanent? What are the alternatives? What do you stand to gain? What are the facts?

We all accept and reject risks every day. Generally, we don't take the time to review data or do a risk/benefit analysis. Think about driving a car. In the US, about 45,000 people die every year in automobile accidents. All of those deaths could be avoided if everyone stopped driving. The risk of death or injury would literally drop to zero. But of course no one is about to trade in his car for a horse. In other words, those of us who drive have determined that the risk of injury or death is acceptable. We need our cars; the benefits outweigh the risks. Within the population of drivers, some people will take on more risky behavior than others. Some will speed; others will drive drunk. But all of us have made some mental calculation as to what is acceptable and the benefits of taking certain risks.

The notion of acceptable risk or benefit is not easy to define. Acceptable risk is essentially the measure of harm or disease that is considered acceptable by a person or a group. Whether a risk is acceptable depends upon the benefits derived from taking the risk, the magnitude of the risk, the available scientific evidence, and various economic, political, and social factors.

We tend to rely on others when we have to determine acceptable health risks, be they risks from exposure to contaminants, or risks and benefits from screening tests and drugs. We often assume that experts in environmental science, biology, medicine, statistics, and other disciplines are more qualified to make decisions as to what constitutes an acceptable health benefit or risk.

Why don't we want to make our own decisions? Largely because there is a prevailing view that acceptable risk values are based on the analysis and interpretation of scientific data and results. But this is simply not the case. Acceptable health risks and benefits are based, in large part, on public acceptance, political agenda, and economic considerations. It may seem counterintuitive, but *there is no science involved in the process.*

Acceptable Environmental Risks

Take the situation, described in Chap. 12, of treating drinking water with chlorine to reduce the likelihood of infections from waterborne contamination. Chlorination is effective in reducing illness from bacteria in water supplies, but potentially carcinogenic chemicals (DBPs) are also formed when chlorine combines with harmless organic compounds naturally present in the water. The EPA had to set the acceptable level of risk resulting from exposure to these chemicals. This federal agency had to determine what constitutes a "safe" level of byproducts from chlorine addition to drinking water. It was a judgment call.

The EPA conducted a risk/benefit analysis and after extensive deliberations picked an acceptable risk level. The Agency considered input from knowledgeable people concerned with this issue. And then they used their best professional judgment. They tried to balance the overall benefits with the overall risks and, to all intents and purposes, their decision was somewhat arbitrary – not driven by scientific information. Another group at a different time with different values and perspectives might have determined that acceptable byproduct levels from chlorine should be higher or lower.

The Federal Safe Drinking Water Act is the law that makes the EPA responsible for regulating chemical substances in drinking water. This legislation allows the EPA some flexibility in determining acceptable risk levels. It allows the EPA to consider the best available control technology.

If chlorination is defined as the most practical and cost effective technology to deal with waterborne contamination, then acceptable risks from chlorination by-products are developed within this context. As a result, the permitted or acceptable risk levels can be less conservative than might be allowed under other environmental legislation.

In drinking water, the acceptable level of cancer risk from DBPs was set at 1 in ten thousand for a lifetime of exposure. Assuming all 300 million Americans were exposed to the maximum allowable levels of carcinogenic chlorinated byproducts in drinking water, it would be acceptable for 30,000 people to get cancer from DBPs over their lifetime.

These same cancer-causing byproducts have an acceptable level of risk of 1 in a million when they occur in rivers, lakes, streams, and oceans – that is, water other than drinking water. Why the difference? Contaminants found in these water bodies are regulated under a different law, the Federal Clean Water Act. The EPA has determined that this legislation mandates a 1 in a million acceptable lifetime risk level for cancer causing substances (i.e., 300 acceptable additional lifetime cancers nationwide). This acceptable risk level is a hundred times more conservative than the 1 in 10,000 acceptable risk level proposed for the addition of chlorine to drinking water.

The EPA must promulgate regulations for both of these laws. Therefore, due to different philosophies, purposes, and objectives, different acceptable levels of risk have been determined for the same contaminant by the same government agency. Scientific information played no role in this process.

Officially, the EPA has adopted a target range for carcinogens of one in ten thousand to one in a million for acceptable risks in different situations. But the EPA and most state and federal agencies usually opt for the more conservative and health protective level of one in a million. In effect, the EPA has determined that the acceptable increase in lifetime risk for exposure to carcinogens in air, soil, sediment, and water (with the exception of drinking water) is one in a million. This acceptable risk level is the principal determinant we have for decisions like what air emissions are allowed or how a hazardous waste site should be cleaned up. In fact, it's difficult to imagine a more widely-used acceptable risk number in the US than the EPA's oft-quoted one in a million risk for lifetime exposure to cancer-causing contaminants.

The risks from exposure to indoor radon and the EPA's policy on this carcinogen (see Chap. 13) provide another example of how acceptable risks and regulatory limits are established. Being a carcinogen, the law assumes that there is no "safe" level of radon. Yet the EPA established the limit on indoor radon levels at 4 pCi/liter. Higher levels are considered excessive, and the EPA recommends that radon controls be implemented for these homes. How did the EPA come to set this limit? In order to determine the acceptable level of radon in indoor air, the Agency had to balance the health risks from exposure to radon, the performance of available methods to fix homes with elevated radon, the number of homes impacted, and the costs involved.

The primary goal of the radon policy is to save lives. The EPA estimates that 450 lives would be saved annually in the US if all of the homes with radon levels above 4 pCi/liter were fixed. For a non-smoker, the risk of cancer from radon exposure at 4 pCi/liter compares to the risk of dying in a car crash. For a smoker, the radon cancer risk is 5 times the risk of dying in a car crash.[1]

As they deliberated the radon limit, the EPA also considered the performance of radon control methods for homes. The most common way to address a radon problem is to seal openings in the foundation and install a vent system. These systems can reduce radon to a level below 2 pCi/liter, which is close to the 1.3 pCi/liter average level of radon in US homes. But these systems cannot reliably achieve background or outdoor radon levels of 0.4 pCi/liter. The EPA had to recognize the practical limits of the available technology.

The EPA could not ignore the economic impacts of the radon limit they were deliberating. The EPA estimates that about one in fifteen homes in the US is likely to have indoor radon levels above 4 pCi/liter. The average installation cost for controlling radon is approximately $1,200.[1] If a limit higher than 4 pCi/liter was selected, then the costs would decrease but fewer lives would be saved. If the limit was lowered, then more lives would be saved but the costs would increase – provided that the available control technologies were able to achieve the lower radon level. In summary, the acceptable indoor air radon level was a compromise between health risks, costs, and the practical limits of being able to fix a radon problem.

Public opinion should also be important in setting an acceptable risk level. Imagine you live in a community of 100,000 people downwind from an incinerator. An investigative reporter has written an article in a well-respected newspaper that outlines the potential health risks from the incinerator's air emissions. In the course of her research, the reporter has found that one of the contaminants, which happens to be a carcinogen, exceeds the EPA's acceptable level of risk. The community's elected officials demand that the EPA conduct a scientific human health risk assessment to confirm or negate her findings. The EPA agrees. In the end, the scientific risk assessment confirms that the measured levels of this pollutant in the air exceed their acceptable level of risk.

The risk assessment results confirm the reporter's calculations. More specifically, this contaminant will result in a risk of 3 in a million. This value is reported to be 200% greater than the EPA's acceptable risk level of 1 in a million. From a relative risk perspective that's an accurate characterization. And in absolute terms, it means that 3 additional people out of a million will die over 70 years from exposure to these contaminants. Since there are only 100,000 residents in your community, this means that 0.3 individuals (about one-third of a person!) are likely to get cancer over the next 70 years. In fact, the EPA uses very conservative, "worst case" assumptions in their risk assessments, and the uncertainty in their calculations is acknowledged to be high, so it's just as likely that the risk will be essentially zero.

The company that runs the incinerator says it cannot afford to lower its emissions. If it has to, it will probably go out of business. EPA remains resolute and emphasizes the importance of not exceeding the acceptable one in a million risk. But Joe Williams, who has a managerial job at the factory and a wife and three kids to support, writes a letter to the EPA telling them that those risks are acceptable to him and to his fellow workers. He tells the EPA that the decision on acceptable risk should be made by the affected community. He tells the governmental agency that this is a value decision, not based on scientific information, and the opinions of people in the community should take precedence over the opinions of those who are not directly impacted.

The EPA responds to Joe, thanking him for his input and explaining that the one in a million value has been around for a very long time; there are sound reasons for using this number. Joe wants to know more about the origin of this widely used risk value. What was the basis and rationale for developing this number? But Joe has trouble finding any written documentation confirming the origin of the acceptable risk level. Indeed, when he contacts representatives of the EPA, FDA, environmental organizations, law firms, state environmental agencies, and other groups, they don't seem to agree on where it came from.

Joe does a little research of his own and finds out that in 1973, the FDA first recommended a level which would represent essentially zero or *de minimus* risk.[2] The term *de minimus* is an abbreviation of the legal concept, *de minimus non curat lex*: the law does not concern itself with trifles. Subsequently, one in a million was developed as the risk cutoff. Anything less was considered a "trifle" and was not of regulatory concern.[3] This decision was prompted by the need to eliminate residues of cancer-causing drugs administered to food-producing animals.

In the FDA legislation, the regulators specifically stated the essentially zero level was not to be interpreted as the same thing as an acceptable level of residues in meat products. This was a critical distinction. But in his research, Joe finds that many current regulations and guidance documents have done exactly that: they have interpreted this essentially zero level as a level which, if exceeded, would represent *an unacceptable risk*. What was intended to be the equivalent of essentially zero risk has been interpreted by many federal and state agencies as a *target level of acceptable risk*.

Given this situation, it would be helpful if the concept of acceptable risk was made more transparent to the public. Informed, involved citizens have a leg to stand on when they demand a voice in determining which risks are and are not acceptable. Then communities could work better with environmental regulators to define acceptable risk in a more equitable and realistic manner.

It is likely that different communities would come up with different levels of acceptable risk. Rather than accepting a one-size-fits-all solution, citizens and local leaders would tailor their risk management decisions to fit the concerns and conditions unique to their community. Since the EPA and state regulatory agencies already support site-specific risk assessments, there is already a precedent for this local approach. Applying the site-specific philosophy to acceptable risk levels increases risk management options across the board.

Acceptable Medical Benefits

When we deal with cancers that don't seem to be caused primarily by exposure to environmental contaminants, then there is no direct analog to the EPA's one in a million acceptable cancer risk level. Nor is there a generally accepted specific value for the number of individuals who would have to benefit to warrant cancer screening tests. That said, encouraging certain segments of the population to be screened for breast, colon, prostate, and other cancers presupposes that worthwhile or acceptable benefits will be derived from these screening programs. These acceptable benefits are no more based on scientific information than is the EPA's one in a million value. By now, it should come as no surprise that they too are based on the values and perspectives of the organizations that manage these health issues.

The purpose of a cancer screening test is to find the cancer when it is still curable, before it becomes established. Do screening tests achieve their objective? To find out, we can compare cancer deaths in a screened group with deaths in a group that has not been screened. Following this line of reasoning, if the benefits of the screening aren't *discernable*, then the merit of the test should be questioned. On the other hand, if the benefit in lives saved turns out to be *meaningful*, then the cost, inconvenience, and potential risk from screening may be worthwhile. In this case, the benefits might be defined as acceptable.

At present, characterizing benefits from cancer screening is a controversial subject. Experts have come to very different recommendations from the same data. In this situation, subjective words like *discernable* and *meaningful* take on considerable importance. For reasons that are not entirely clear, the controversy and uncertainty surrounding the benefits of screening tests have not been effectively communicated to medical patients.

We are inundated with media reports and statements from reputable medical organizations that laud the benefits of screening for cancer. We hear in no uncertain terms that PSA tests, colonoscopies, and mammograms will reduce the incidence of cancer and therefore reduce the number of deaths from this most deadly disease. A recent article reported how death rates for most forms of cancer have continued to decline, including a 1.6 percent annual decline in cancer deaths for men from 1992 to 2003 and a 0.8 percent annual drop among women.[4] One gets the seemingly clear impression that cancer screening is in large part responsible for the decline in cancer deaths.

However, another article reported that "an examination of the annual statistical data compiled by the American Cancer Society quickly reveals that the rate of mortality from cancer has changed very little over the past 50 years."[5] This article appeared only a few months before the other, and yet these two reports on the same human health topic give essentially opposite messages. They illustrate the conflicting information that frequently arises from interpreting and communicating health benefits and risks.

At this point, you may be wondering if the benefits from cancer screening tests are as pronounced as media reports make them sound. Is there agreement in the medical community that these tests will result in an acceptable reduction in cancer mortality? If not, why are millions of people throughout the world taking the time, accepting the risks involved, and paying for these tests? Somehow, asking these questions can even feel inappropriate in the current climate of widespread acceptance for these screening tests.

But the questions are legitimate. At present, the National Cancer Institute (NCI) is sponsoring a major cancer clinical trial involving more than 155,000 men and women.[6] The primary objective is "... to determine if certain cancer screening practices reduce the number of deaths from prostate, lung, colon and ovarian cancer." In other words, in the year 2006, evidence is still insufficient to determine whether there are acceptable death benefits from the cancer screening tests that are recommended to millions of patients throughout the world. Of the four cancer screening tests that will be evaluated in the NCI study, only colon cancer screening has been shown to reduce the number of deaths (see Chap. 10). To date, there is not yet clear evidence that prostate, ovarian, and lung cancer screening tests have any benefits in terms of reduced mortality.

The lack of evidence could simply mean that a long term clinical study hasn't been undertaken. There could still be anecdotal reasons to believe that screening tests are very effective. And without other viable alternatives, why not use this anecdotal information to encourage people to take these screening tests? Future research may confirm the health benefits from screening for certain cancers, and then we'll be glad we've been doing screening all along. But even if the benefits aren't confirmed, what harm could come from screening?

But with screening tests, there is the possibility for both false positives and false negatives. A false positive result suggests the patient has the disease when in fact, he doesn't. Imagine the anxiety, not to mention the further tests and treatment which are unnecessary. On the other hand, a false negative result suggests the disease is not present, when in fact the patient has the disease. He could benefit from medical attention, but doesn't know to seek help. False positives and negatives contribute to uncertainty in determining the effectiveness of screening tests.

As a specific example of the uncertainty associated with acceptable screening benefits, let's consider prostate cancer. The American Cancer Society estimates that there will be approximately 235,000 new cases of prostate cancer in the US and approximately 27,000 deaths in 2006.[7] This cancer is the most common cancer among men, with the exception of skin cancer. Due to the prevalence and seriousness of the disease, considerable effort has gone into developing a screening test. The recommended prostate cancer screen (see Chap. 7) continues to be a controversial subject of passionate debate in the medical community.[8,9]

Medical experts differ on the value and appropriateness of prostate cancer screening. At present, the American Cancer Society and the American Urological Association support the use of PSA and DRE screening beginning at age 50 in normal-risk men. On the other hand, the American Medical Association and the American College of Physicians – American Society for Internal Medicine do not recommend prostate cancer screening.[10] And the United States Preventative Services Task Force decided that the net benefit of prostate cancer screening with PSA and DRE could not be determined.[11]

In 2005, an article was published in the Journal of the National Cancer Institute regarding prostate cancer screening. This article discussed the status of prostate cancer screening as part of the NCI-sponsored PLCO (e.g., prostate, lung, colon, ovarian) cancer screening trial:

The benefit of screening for prostate cancer using prostate-specific antigen (PSA) testing and digital rectal examination (DRE) is uncertain and is under evaluation in a randomized prospective trial, the Prostate, Lung, Colorectal and Ovarian (PLCO) Cancer Screening Trial. Although the final results are several years away, the initial round of screening is complete.

The PLCO trial is evaluating PSA- and DRE-based screening for prostate cancer in a clinically valid manner. Whether such screening will result in a reduction of prostate cancer mortality cannot be answered until the randomized comparison is completed.[12]

So what's the bottom line? Currently, there doesn't seem to be evidence that screening results in the reduction of prostate cancer mortality. Experts disagree as to whether or not to recommend this screen. In terms of acceptable benefits, the verdict is not yet in. But what if your doctor tells you your DRE and PSA level suggests the need for a biopsy? What if you agree and the biopsy is positive? Knowing the risks (impotence, infection, and incontinence), do you go ahead with surgery? What if the cancer is the slow-growing kind that may not affect your health? You will have to face these difficult questions.

There are also more general questions which need to be asked. Shouldn't patients be informed of the considerable controversy among scientists and physicians regarding screening test benefits? The very existence of this major NCI study supports the argument that evidence on death benefits is currently lacking. Lack of evidence is not something that we should dismiss summarily. But if your doctor strongly recommends screening based on her assessment of anecdotal evidence, on what basis would you disagree with her recommendation? Then again, historical precedent suggests that we should view strong and definitive recommendations supporting the use of cancer screening tests and drugs with caution.

Having the proper data available in a user-friendly format will enable each of us to determine the level of benefits and risks which we can accept. We have a right to this information, and an acknowledgement of this right will serve to empower patients and citizens. But if we want solid answers to legitimate questions, we must engage and participate in the entire process.

If you want to determine your own level of acceptable risk you can't rely on professionals speculating about "what the public wants." You must be proactive and demand relevant information in order to participate legitimately in decisions about acceptable benefits and risks. In order to win a voice, it will require persistence and hard work.

Everyone concerned with this issue must contend with uncertainties inherent to even the best risk and benefit assessments. Uncertainties are often especially large where risks and benefits are small. Acknowledging, accepting, and understanding this uncertainty would be a critical and important first step. While coming to grips with uncertainty may be difficult for health professionals and the public alike, it would go a long way toward removing the illusion of certainty which currently exists.

Appendices

Appendix A: A Brief Primer on Statistical Approaches for Quantifying Uncertainty

The many sources of uncertainty in characterizing health benefits and risks are discussed in Chap. 5. A simple way to communicate uncertainty is to use statistical tools to convey the nature of the distribution of possible risks or benefits.[1,2] First off, what is this *distribution*? If we want to estimate the risk of cancer from exposure to pulp mill air emissions, we have to consider all the uncertainty discussed in Chaps. 4 and 5. We have to consider a case for children and another for adults, one for sick people, and another for healthy people. Different weather patterns will mean different exposures; we'll have to consider a case for each. The amount of dioxin in the emissions varies depending on how the pulp mill is operating, so we'll have to consider a few different cases for the amount of dioxin released. And just how dangerous is the dioxin, anyway? Different labs reported different results from animal studies, and different models gave different estimates for low dose extrapolation. We will come up with a different risk estimate for each combination and permutation. This set of estimates is our distribution of possible risks.

Mean and Standard Deviation

It's unwieldy to deal with the entire distribution of numbers. So we want to summarize the risks in a form that is easier to understand. First, we might ask, "considering all the various cases, what's the typical risk; what's normal?" This answer is one single number, called the *mean* or *arithmetic average*, and it's a convenient summary. Ok, but how normal is normal? Across all our different combinations and situations, do we always come up with a similar estimate of risk? Or are the results spread all over the place? In other words, what is the *variation* in the results? The simplest way to describe the variation is by reporting the *range* of our estimates, or the spread from the minimum to the maximum. But statisticians prefer a more powerful measure called the *standard deviation* of the data. Every risk estimate will be a little different; they can't all be exactly "normal." The standard deviation answers the question, "on average, how far are these risk estimates from normal, how different are they from the mean?" If all our risk estimates are very similar for all of our different situations, they will all be quite close to the "typical" mean, the standard deviation will be small, and we will be more confident that we have a good estimate of the risk: the uncertainty will be lower. Example calculations using these statistical tools to convey uncertainty are given in the following section.

Example Calculations: a hypothetical case study

The mean or arithmetic average of data, $\overline{X}$, is computed using the following equation:

$$\overline{X} = \frac{\sum_{i=1}^{N} X_i}{N}.$$ (Eq. 1)

X_i is the ith data value among a series of N numbers, and N is the total number of data values. The symbol $\sum$ means to sum or add all the X_i values. The standard deviation of the data, s, is calculated using the following equation:

$$s = \sqrt{\frac{\sum_{i=1}^{N}(X_i - \overline{X})^2}{N-1}}.$$ (Eq. 2)

The following case study illustrates how these equations can be used to interpret exposure and associated health risks. Quarterly samples collected from a water well are analyzed for "Chemical X" for two years to provide information on the drinking water concentrations for this compound. The hypothetical concentration data appear in Table A.1.

Table A.1. Hypothetical concentrations of Chemical X in well water

Sample Period	Concentration, $\mu g/L^a$	Sample Period	Concentration, $\mu g/L^*$
1st quarter	12	5th quarter	6
2nd quarter	3	6th quarter	9
3rd quarter	4	7th quarter	10
4th quarter	7	8th quarter	2

[a] The concentration unit of $\mu g/L$ stands for microgram per liter and is the same as one millionth of a gram per liter.

The mean concentration is calculated using Eq. 1 and is 6.6 $\mu g/L$. The standard deviation is calculated by using Eq. 2 and is 3.5 $\mu g/L$. The common way to express these results is 6.6 ± 3.5 $\mu g/L$. The uncertainty in the average value represents the time variation in Chemical X concentration that is influenced by geological variation and the errors associated with sample collection and laboratory analysis. The amount of variability shown in this example calculation is typically observed during groundwater monitoring efforts.

Chemical X is a carcinogen, and several health experts are asked to determine the lifetime risk of developing cancer if this water is used for drinking. Animal toxicity studies with Chemical X are costly and time consuming, so there are only four health studies available for this carcinogen. The hypothetical lifetime cancer risk data are shown below.

Health Expert 1: Risk is 1/1,000,000 or 0.000001
Health Expert 2: Risk is 1/20,000 or 0.00005
Health Expert 3: Risk is 1/50,000,000 or 0.00000002
Health Expert 4: Risk is 1/100,000 or 0.00001

The mean cancer risk and standard deviation calculated from Eqs. 1 and 2 are 0.000015 ± 0.000024. Note that a risk approaching zero falls within the one standard deviation risk interval. The one standard deviation range for the cancer risk is zero to 1/25,600.

Sensitivity Analysis

The next level of complexity in formal uncertainty analysis is to perform a sensitivity analysis. Usually, it's not obvious which assumptions and uncertainties most significantly affect the conclusions. So the purpose of sensitivity analysis is to find out which parameters or inputs are likely to have significant effects on model outputs or predictions. Experience has shown that in most cases, a relatively small subset of variables is influential. Estimates of the variability in the influential parameters and inputs are then carried through the model to improve the confidence in the model predictions that are applied to a specific situation.

Another approach to evaluating uncertainty is to use probabilistic techniques that have been developed over the past decade or two. These methods consider a range of numbers to provide more realistic exposure data and risk assessments. These techniques replace point estimates with distributions for important exposure parameters so that the results reflect the range and probability of the possible outcomes. One common probabilistic technique is Monte Carlo analysis (described in Box A.1). Probabilistic approaches are considered to be optimal for characterizing exposure and health risks, because they do not tend to result in overly-conservative or non-plausible risk values.

Box A.1. Monte Carlo Simulation

Virtually every variable in exposure assessment, whether physiological, behavioral, environmental, or chronological can be replaced with a probability distribution. The steps in running a Monte Carlo simulation for an exposure analysis include:[3]

1. The probability distribution of each input parameter is characterized and specified (or a random selection of input data).
2. For each iteration of the simulation, one value is randomly selected from each parameter distribution, and the equation/model is run. Many iterations are performed, such that the random selections for each parameter approximate the distributions of the parameter. Five-thousand or more iterations are typically performed.
3. Each iteration is evaluated and saved so a probability distribution of the equation output is generated. This distribution reflects the likely range of outcomes for the specific situation being assessed.

Even in this short summary and example, the technical details of calculating and representing uncertainty with numbers become complicated. As noted in Chaps. 3 and 5, the risk characterization theater (RCT) can be a useful graphic to visualize the range of possible numbers. Multiple RCTs can illustrate the uncertainty associated with the chance of a benefit or risk by showing a range of likely outcomes. If the necessary information is available, health benefit and risk numbers should be expressed not as a single value but as a range of values. For the interested reader, several references are available on the topic of statistics and other mathematical tools for uncertainty analysis.[4,5,6]

Appendix B: Two Clinical Studies that Evaluated Blood Serum Cholesterol as a Risk Factor for Coronary Heart Disease (CHD)

Chapter 8 provides an analysis of elevated cholesterol as a primary risk factor for heart disease. The purpose for this appendix is to provide an expanded discussion of the clinical studies referenced in Chap. 8.

The best-known clinical study attempting to correlate blood serum cholesterol levels and the incidence of CHD is the Framingham Study.[1] This study, which began in 1948, was supported by the National Heart, Lung, and Blood Institute and involved some 5,000 men and women from a Boston suburb. These individuals were followed, examined, and reported on at intervals for more than 50 years to determine if there was an association between serum blood cholesterol levels and CHD. One outcome of the Framingham study is a comparison of blood serum cholesterol in men who did not have CHD (termed "CHD-Free Men" in the study) and men who developed CHD (Fig. B.1). These data show that many men who developed CHD had cholesterol levels between 140 and 220 mg/100 ml – a range that is frequently considered to be essentially normal. Furthermore, the distribution of cholesterol levels among men who did not have CHD and those who did develop CHD is fairly close.

According to the Framingham data in Fig. B.1, 100% of the men in the two study groups had a mean serum cholesterol level at or below 460 mg/100 ml. Using this as a reference, another way to represent the data shown in Fig. B.1 is to determine the percentage of men in the two study groups whose mean serum cholesterol was at or below a specific level. A new plot in Fig. B.2 shows this summed distribution. In this manner, the intersection of the 50% point and each curve represents the cholesterol level that is exactly in the middle of each study group. The advantage of this new plot (Fig. B.2) is that the cholesterol level corresponding to the middle of each study group (the 50% point) can be more readily obtained. For the men with CHD, the 50% point corresponds to a cholesterol level of 220 mg/100 ml. This means that just as many men developed CHD with cholesterol levels below 220 mg/100 ml as did those with cholesterol levels above 220 mg/100 ml. In other words, the two groups of men who had blood serum cholesterol levels above or below 220 mg/100 ml – a level that is frequently stated as the line between elevated and essentially normal levels – developed CHD at about the same rate.

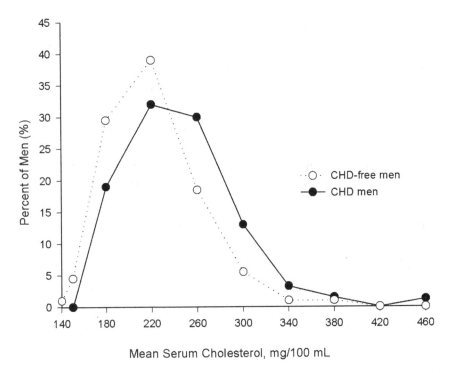

Mean Serum Cholesterol, mg/100 mL

Fig. B.1. Distribution of serum cholesterol in subjects free of coronary heart disease versus those developing coronary heart disease in 16 years; men aged 30 to 49 years at entry. Data from the Framingham Study[1]

The largest and most comprehensive clinical study on cholesterol levels and heart disease is the Multiple Risk Factor Intervention Trial, or MRFIT.[2,3] In this second clinical study, over 350,000 male participants had their cholesterol levels measured and monitored for 6 years. Shown in Fig. B.3 is the summed distribution of cholesterol levels in men without CHD and in men who died from CHD, based on data from MRFIT. The blood serum cholesterol level where 50% of the population died from CHD virtually duplicates the results obtained from the Framingham study (in the case of MRFIT, the 50% level is 225 mg/100 ml). The MRFIT data indicate that the two groups of men who had blood serum cholesterol levels below or above 225 mg/100 ml died at about the same rate.

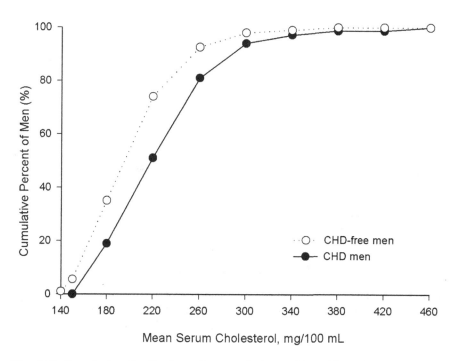

Fig. B.2. Cumulative distribution of serum cholesterol in subjects free of coronary heart disease versus those developing coronary heart disease in 16 years; men aged 30 to 49 years at entry. Data from the Framingham Study[1]

In both Figs. B.2 and B.3, the respective curves for participants with CHD and dying from CHD are shifted slightly to the right. One reason for the shift is that both cholesterol levels and the incidence of CHD increase with age.[4] It is hard to adjust the data to account for these variables. Another possible reason for the shift is that those with CHD at the higher cholesterol levels shown in the figures are likely to include participants with diabetes, a genetic disorder (familial hypercholesteremia), and other diseases. People with these diseases have a higher risk of dying from CHD and do not appear to be excluded from the analysis.

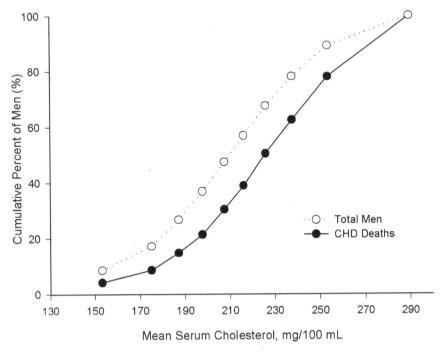

Fig. B.3. Cumulative distribution of serum cholesterol in subjects free of coronary heart disease at the start of the study versus those who died from coronary heart disease in 6 years; men aged 35-57 at entry. Data from the MRFIT study[3]

Appendix C: Glossary

Absolute risk – Your risk of developing a disease over a specified period of time. It reflects the number of people who will get the disease, *compared to the total number of people being considered*. For example, if 6 people out of 100 will get the disease, then the absolute risk is 6 / 100 = 0.06. It can also be expressed as a 6% absolute risk or a 6 in 100 absolute risk.

Absolute risk reduction (ARR) – This is the difference between two absolute risks in two groups. For example, let's say that 6 people out of 100 (6%) get a certain kind of liver disease and die from it. An effective new drug is invented; when people take this drug, only 4 out of 100 (4%) get this liver disease and die from it. So the absolute risk reduction is 6% – 4% = 2%. In other words, 2 lives are saved out of 100. ARR compares the number of people who will benefit from intervention (in this case, 2) to the *total number of people being considered* (in this case, 100)

Acceptable medical benefit – The measure of benefit that is considered acceptable by a person or group. It is generally based on values, perceptions, views, and opinions.

Acceptable risk level – The measure of harm or disease that is considered acceptable by a person or group. It is generally based on values, perceptions, views, and opinions.

Atherosclerosis – A chronic cardiovascular disease characterized by the deposition of plaques containing lipids, cells, cholesterol, and other substances on the innermost layer of the walls of certain arteries.

Average – The value obtained by dividing the sum of a set of quantities by the number of quantities in the set.

Biomarker – A distinctive and detectable substance which is naturally present in the body and can be used as an indicator of a certain biological process, event, or condition. For example, elevated PSA is used as a biomarker for prostate cancer.

Cancer – An abnormal growth of cells which tend to proliferate in uncontrolled ways and, in some cases, spread (metastasize).

Carcinogen – A chemical or other agent known or believed to cause cancer. The number of known human carcinogens is relatively small but many chemicals and agents are suspected of being carcinogens.

Cardiovascular disease – A general category consisting of several separate diseases of the heart and circulatory system. The two most important components are coronary heart disease and stroke.

Cause and effect – Refers to a relationship whereby an agent (cause) must be present if an effect is to occur. In the context of human health, the agent is responsible for a disease (e.g., HIV is the cause, AIDS is the effect).

Chlorination – A common and effective process where chlorine is used to destroy pathogenic bacteria and other harmful agents; particularly used to disinfect drinking water.

Cholesterol – A waxy substance present in blood serum and in all animal tissues. Cholesterol is essential to life and is a component of the membrane that surrounds animal cells. It is also associated with plaque formed in arteries. The concentration of cholesterol in your blood is called "blood serum cholesterol." Blood serum cholesterol is measured in milligrams per 100 milliliters, often abbreviated as "mg."

Chromium – A metallic element used in the hardening of steel alloys and the production of stainless steel. In the environment, it can be found as both toxic and non-toxic forms.

Coronary heart disease – Progressive reduction of the blood supply to the heart due to a narrowing or blocking of a coronary artery.

Disinfection by-products – Compounds formed at a water treatment plant when chlorine is added to water that contains organic material. Some of these by-products can be carcinogens.

Distribution – A set of numbers and their frequency of occurrence collected from measurements in a population.

Dose-response assessment – This quantitative step in the risk assessment process is designed to determine the relationship between the amount of a chemical or substance present and the incidence of an adverse health effect.

Ecological risk assessment – A scientific approach used to determine the possible impacts of human activities on the environment. This process evaluates the likelihood that adverse ecological effects may occur from exposure to contaminants or other modifications to ecosystems.

Ecosystem – A functional system that includes an ecological community of organisms together with the physical environment interacting as a unit.

Environmental contaminant – A substance that is responsible for polluting and degrading the quality of soil, air, sediment, or water resources.

Epidemiological study – A population study designed to examine associations between personal characteristics and environmental exposures that may increase the risk of disease.

Exposure assessment – This quantitative step in the risk assessment process involves determining the number of people exposed and the magnitude and duration of the exposure to a contaminant present in the environment.

Hazard identification – This qualitative step in the risk assessment process involves evaluating data on the kinds of health effects that occur after exposure to an environmental insult.

Lifetime – For the purpose of estimating "lifetime" cancer risks, the EPA sets the human lifetime at 70 years. "Lifetime" data reported by other organizations may refer to a longer or shorter time period. In the medical discussions in this book, the word is also used generally to describe long-term risks or benefits.

No observable adverse effect level – A threshold concentration for non-carcinogens below which there is assumed to be no harmful (adverse) effect. The NOAEL is usually established from experimental data with test organisms.

Number needed to treat – The number of people who must undergo medical treatment or screening in order for one person to benefit.

Order of magnitude – A factor of ten; ten times. For example, the number 1,002 is about an order of magnitude bigger than the number 99.

Pathogen – An agent that causes infection or disease. Example pathogens include certain bacteria, protozoa, and viruses.

Peer review – Process where a researcher's work is examined and criticized by experts in the field before it is approved for publication. Peer review adds credibility.

Plaque – A fatty deposit on the innermost layer of an artery wall; characteristic of atherosclerosis.

Population – A group of individuals (or animals, etc.) who can be studied as a whole because they have something in common that is relevant for the analysis.

Primary prevention – Activities or measures that help avoid a given health care problem. Effective primary prevention helps keep you from getting sick in the first place.

Prostate-specific antigen – A protein produced in the prostate gland that appears in the blood; elevated levels are used as an indicator of prostate cancer in diagnostic screening tests.

Radon – A colorless, radioactive gas formed by the radioactive decay of radium. Radon occurs in minute amounts in soil, rocks, and the air near the ground.

Relative risk reduction (RRR) – Reflects the number of people who benefit from an intervention, *compared to the number of people who get the disease if they aren't treated* (but not compared to the total number of people being considered). Thus RRR measures how much the risk is reduced in the experimental group compared to a control group, and is calculated as the ratio of two absolute risk numbers. It is almost always expressed in percent. When results are expressed as a relative risk reduction, the absolute risk levels for the experimental and control groups are not known. For example, if taking a new drug reduces the number of liver disease deaths from 6 out of 100 (6%) to 4 out of 100 (4%), then the relative risk reduction is 33 percent because 4% is 33 percent less than 6%. So we could say that the drug cuts your chances of dying of this liver disease by 33 percent, or else that you are only two-thirds as likely to die of the disease if you take the drug.

Risk – The possibility of experiencing some sort of harm, loss, or other negative effect. Risk is ubiquitous. In the context of this book, we are concerned with risk associated with the medical conditions and treatments we may endure and the exposure we may have to environmental contaminants. Conversely, the possibility of experiencing a positive effect is called a chance of benefit.

Risk assessment – An evaluation of the likelihood of adverse human health and ecological effects that may result from exposure to certain hazards, especially environmental contaminants. The same principles are also used to evaluate the benefits from medical screening tests and drugs.

Risk characterization – The integration of information on hazard, dose-response, and exposure to develop quantitative estimates of risk and to determine the uncertainties associated with the risk estimate. Risk characterization integrates quantitative and qualitative elements.

Risk characterization theater – A graphic developed by the authors that uses a theater with a seating capacity of 1,000 to illustrate the number of individuals who would benefit from a medical intervention or be impacted by exposure to an environmental contaminant. Imagine yourself sitting in this theater. In the crowd that surrounds you, certain people will benefit from the treatment being discussed, or in a different example, they will be harmed by the disease at hand. Sometimes, you yourself will be affected.

In the RCT diagram, these affected people are represented by darkened seats.

Risk communication – The process of exchanging information among individuals, groups, and institutions about the nature of a risk value.

Risk factor – A biological condition, substance, or behavior that has an association with but has not been proven to cause an event or disease.

Risk management – A political activity that balances interests and values to determine whether human health risks should be considered tolerable or unacceptable.

Screening test – The primary purpose of this medical intervention is to identify disease in people who don't yet have symptoms of the illness.

Secondary prevention – Activities or measures that involve the care of an established disease. Secondary prevention attempts to minimize the negative effects of the disease and avoid disease-related complications in people who already have the disease.

Standard deviation – In statistics, a measure of how much the data in a grouping of results are scattered around the average value. A low standard deviation means that the data are tightly clustered; a high standard deviation means that the data are widely scattered.

Statins – Any of a class of lipid-lowering drugs that reduce blood serum cholesterol levels by inhibiting a key enzyme involved in the biosynthesis of cholesterol. Known lipid-independent effects of statins include reduction of inflammatory cells, reduced levels of C-reactive protein, and inhibition of platelet aggregation.

Stroke – The sudden death of a portion of the brain due to a lack of oxygen. The lack of oxygen is often due to some sort of blockage in the circulatory system. Stroke can cause parts of the brain to function abnormally.

Uncertainty – The lack of assurance in the numerical value of a health benefit or risk.

References

Chapter 1

1. Zehr SC (1999) Scientists' representations of uncertainty. In: Friedman SM, Dunwoody S, Rogers CL (eds) Communicating uncertainty - media coverage of new and controversial science. Lawrence Erlbaum Associates, Publishers, London, 277 pp.
2. Gawande A (2002) Complications - a surgeon's notes on an imperfect science. Picador Publishers, New York, 269 pp.
3. Carson R (1962) Silent Spring. Houghton Mifflin Co., New York, 300 pp.
4. Ruckelshaus WD (1983) Science, risk, and public policy. Science 221(4615): 1026-1028.

Chapter 2

1. Lave LB (1987) Health and safety risk analyses: information for better decisions. Science 236(4799):291-295.
2. Gotzsche PC, Olsen O (2000) Is screening for breast cancer with mammography justifiable? The Lancet 355(9198):129-134.
3. Fisher B, Constantino JP, Wickerham DL, Redmond CK, Kavanah M, Cronin WM, Vogel V, Robidous A, Dimitrov N, Atkins J, Daly M, Wieand S, Tan-Chiu E, Ford L, Wolmark N (1998) Tamoxifen for prevention of breast cancer: report of the National Surgical Adjuvant Breast and Bowel Project P-1 Study. J Natnl Cancer Inst 90(18):1371-1388.
4. Mansley EC, McKenna MT (2001) Importance of perspective in economic analyses of cancer screening decisions. The Lancet 358(9288):1169-1173.

Chapter 3

1. Russell C (1986) The View from the national beat. In: Friedman SM, Dunwoody S, Rogers CL (eds) Scientists and journalists: reporting science as news. Published for the American Association for the Advancement of Science by the Free Press, Macmillan, New York City, 333 pp.

2. Hochhauser M, Goldfarb NM (2005) (Mis)Communicating COX-2 clinical trial results. (Accessed July 2006); http://www.firstclinical.com.
3. Elting LS, Martin CG, Cantor SB, Rosenthal EB (1999) Influence of data display formats on physician investigators' decisions to stop clinical trials: prospective trial with repeated measures. BMJ 318:1527-1531.

Chapter 4

1. Ruckelshaus WD (1983) Science, risk, and public policy. Science 221(4615): 1026-1028.
2. Goldstein B (1985) Risk assessment and risk management of benzene by the Environmental Protection Agency. In: Hoel DG, Merrill RA, Revera FP (eds) Banbury Report 19: Risk quantification and regulatory policy. Cold Spring Harbor Laboratory, New York, pp. 293-304.
3. U.S. Environmental Protection Agency (US EPA) (1984) National emission standards for hazardous air pollutants; regulation of benzene; response to public comments. Federal Register 49(23):478-493.
4. Raffensperger C, Tickner J (eds) (1999) Protecting public health and the environment: implementing the precautionary principle. Island Press, Washington, D.C., 385 pp.
5. Leape J (1980) Quantitative risk assessment in regulation of environmental carcinogens. Harv Environ Law Rev 4(86):86-116.
6. Latin H (1997) Science, regulation, and toxic risk assessment. In: Molak V (ed.) Fundamentals of risk analysis and risk management. CRC press, Boca Raton, FL, pp. 303-323.
7. U.S. EPA (1986) Risk assessment guidelines of 1986, EPA/600/8-82/045, August 1987.
8. Kurland L, Faro S, Siedler H (1960) Minamata disease. World Neurol 1:320-325.
9. NRC (National Research Council, U.S.) (2001) A risk-management strategy for PCB-contaminated sediments. National Academy Press, Washington, D.C., 452 pp.
10. NRC (National Research Council, U.S.) (1983) Risk assessment in the federal government: managing the process. National Academy Press, Washington, D.C., 191 pp.
11. Calabrese EJ (1987) Animal extrapolation: a look inside the toxicologist's black box. Environ Sci Tech 21(7):618-623.

Chapter 5

1. Morgan MG, Henrion M (1990) Uncertainty: a guide to dealing with uncertainty in quantitative risk and policy analysis. Cambridge University Press, Cambridge, England, 332 pp.

2. Slovic P (2002) Trust, emotion, sex, politics, and science: surveying the risk-assessment battlefield (Ch. 27). In: Paustenbach DJ (ed) Human and ecological risk assessment: theory and practice. Wiley-Interscience, New York City, pp. 1377-1397.

3. Wiener JB (2002) Precaution in a multirisk world (Ch. 32). In: Paustenbach DJ (ed) Human and ecological risk assessment: theory and practice. Wiley-Interscience, New York City, pp. 1509-1531.

4. Williams PRD, Paustenbach DJ (2002) Risk characterization (Ch. 5). In: Paustenbach DJ (ed) Human and ecological risk assessment: theory and practice. Wiley-Interscience, New York City, pp. 293-366.

5. Gold LS, Ames BN, Slone TH (2002) Misconceptions about the causes of cancer (Ch. 29). In: Paustenbach DJ (ed) Human and ecological risk assessment: theory and practice. Wiley-Interscience, New York City, pp. 1415-1460.

6. U.S. EPA (1985) Principles of risk assessment: a nontechnical review. Prepared by Environ Corporation for a risk assessment workshop, Easton, MD, March 17-18.

7. National Research Council (NRC) (1983) Risk assessment in the federal government: managing the process. National Academy Press, Washington, D.C., 191 pp.

8. Calabrese EJ (1987) Animal extrapolation: a look inside the toxicologist's black box. Environ Sci Tech 21(7): 618-623.

9. Paustenbach DJ (2002) Exposure assessment (Ch. 4), In: Paustenbach DJ (ed) Human and ecological risk assessment: theory and practice. Wiley-Interscience, New York City, pp. 189-291.

10. National Research Council (NRC) (1999) Environmental cleanup at navy facilities. National Academy Press, Washington, D.C., 143 pp.

11. Hattis D (2004) The conception of variability in risk analysis: developments since 1980, In: McDaniels T, Small MJ (eds) Risk analysis and society: an interdisciplinary characterization of the field. Cambridge University Press, Cambridge, United Kingdom, pp. 15-45.

12. National Research Council (1993) Issues in risk assessment. National Academies Press, Washington, D.C., 374 pp.

13. Sergeant A (2002) Ecological risk assessment: history and fundamentals (Ch. 6). In: Paustenbach DJ (ed) Human and ecological risk assessment: theory and practice. Wiley-Interscience, New York City, pp. 369-442.

14. Cullen AC, Small MJ (2004) Uncertain risk: the role and limits of quantitative assessment. In: McDaniels T, Small MJ (eds) Risk analysis and society: an interdisciplinary characterization of the field. Cambridge University Press, Cambridge, United Kingdom, pp. 163-212.

15. Ramaswami A, Milford JB, Small, MJ (2005) Integrated environmental modeling: pollutant transport, fate, and risk in the environment. John Wiley and Sons, Inc., Hoboken, NJ, 678 pp.
16. Wilson R, Crouch EAC (1987) Risk assessment and comparisons: an introduction. Science 236(4799):267-270.
17. Thompson KM, Bloom DL (2000) Communication of risk assessment information to risk managers. J Risk Research 3(4):333-352.
18. Hogue C (2006) Changes for research at EPA. Chemical and Engineering News 84(20):38-41.

Chapter 6

1. Solomon DH, Avorn J (2005) Coxibs, science, and the public trust, an editorial. Arch Intern Med 165:158-160.
2. Graham DJ, Campen D, Hui R, Spence M, Cheetham C, Levy G, Shoor S, Ray WA (2005) Risk of acute myocardial infarction and sudden cardiac death in patients treated with cyclo-oxygenase 2 selective and non-selective non-steroidal anti-inflammatory drugs: nested case-control study. The Lancet 365(9458):475-481.
3. Dai C, Stafford RS, Alexander GC (2005) National trends in cyclooxygenase-2 inhibitor use since market release, Nonselective diffusion of a selectively cost-effective innovation. Arch Intern Med 165(2):171-177.
4. Green GA (2001) Understanding NSAIDs: from aspirin to COX-2. Clin Cornerstone 3(5):50-59
5. Silverstein FE, Faich G, Goldstein JL, Simon LS, Pincus T, Whelton A, Makuch R, Eisen G, Agrawal NM, Stenson WF, Burr AM, Zhao WW, Kent JD, Lefkowith JB, Verburg, KM, Geis GS (2000) Gastrointestinal toxicity with celecoxib vs. nonsteroidal anti-inflammatory drugs for osteoarthritis and rheumatoid arthritis: The CLASS study: a randomized controlled trial. JAMA 284(10):1247-1255.
6. Bombardier C, Laine L, Reicin A, Shapiro D, Burgos-Vargas R, Davis B, Day R, Bosi Ferraz M, Hawkey CJ, Hochberg MC, Kvien TK, Schnitzer TJ for the VIGOR Study Group (2000) Comparison of upper gastrointestinal toxicity of rofecoxib and naproxen in patients with rheumatoid arthritis. N Engl J Med 343(21):1520-1528.
7. Hochhauser M, Goldfarb NM (2005) (Mis) Communicating COX-2 clinical trial results. (Accesed July 2006); http://www.firstclinical.com

Chapter 7

1. Andriole GL, Levin DL, Crawford ED, Gelmann EP, Pinsky PF, Chia D, Kramer BS, Reding D, Church TR, Grubb, RL, Izmirlian G, Ragard LR, Clapp JD, Prorok PC, Gohagan JK, PLCO Project Team (2005) Prostate cancer screening in the prostate, lung, colorectal and ovarian (PLCO) cancer

screening trial: findings from the initial screening round of a randomized trial. J Nat Can Instit 97(6):433-438.

2. Surveillance, Epidemiology, and End Results (SEER) Program (May 1997) Public use CD-ROM (1973-94) by the National Cancer Institute, DCPC, Surveillance Program, Cancer Statistics Branch.

3. U.S. Preventive Services Task Force (1996) Guide to Clinical Preventive Services, 2nd ed. Lippincott Williams & Wilkins, Baltimore, 953 pp.

4. Thompson IM, Pauler DK, Goodman PJ, Tangen CM, Lucia MS, Parnes HL, Minasian LM, Ford LG, Lippman SM, Crawford ED, Crowley JJ, Coltman CA (2004) Prevalence of prostate cancer among men with a prostate-specific antigen level < 4.0 g per milliliter. New Engl J Med 350(22):2239-2246.

5., Lefevre ML, (1998) Prostate cancer screening: more harm than good? American Family Physician 58(2):432-438.

6. Keetch DW, Catalona WJ, Smith DS (1994) Serial prostatic biopsies in men with persistently elevated serum prostate specific antigen values. J Urol 151(6):1571-1574.

7. Ries LAG, Eisner MP, Kosary CL, Hanke BF, Miller BA, Clegg L, Mariotto A, Feuer EJ, Edwards BK (eds) (2004) SEER cancer statistics review, 1975-2001. National Cancer Institute, Bethesda, MD, (available online at http://seer.cancer.gov/csr/1975-2001).

8. Eichler K, Wilby J, Hempel S, Myers L, Kleijnen J (2005) Diagnostic value of systematic prostate biopsy methods in the investigation for prostate cancer: a systematic review (CRD Report 29). University of York, York, 215 pp.

Chapter 8

1. Ravnskov U (2000) The cholesterol myths. New Trends Publishing, Inc., Washington, D.C., 305 pp.

2. American Heart Association (2006) Heart disease and stroke statistics – 2006 update. Circulation 113(6):e85-151.

3. Expert Panel on Detection, Evaluation, and Treatment of High Blood Cholesterol in Adults (2001) Executive summary of the third report of the National Cholesterol Education Program (NCEP) Expert Panel on Detection, Evaluation, and Treatment of High Blood Cholesterol in Adults (Adults Treatment Panel III). JAMA 285(19):2486-2497.

4. Ridker PM (2003) High-sensitivity C-reactive protein and cardiovascular risk: rationale for screening and primary prevention. Amer J Card 92(4 supp 2):17K-22K.

5. DeBakey ME, Glaeser DH (2000) Patterns of atherosclerosis: effect of risk factors on recurrence and survival – analysis of 11,890 cases with more than 25-year follow-up. Amer J Card 85(9):1045-1053.

6. Kannel WB, Dawber TR, Friedman GD, Glennon WE, McNamara PM (1964) Risk factors in coronary heart disease: an evaluation of several serum lipids as

predictors of coronary heart disease; The Framingham Study. Ann Intern Med 61:888-899.

7. Castelli WP, Anderson K (1986) A population at risk: Prevalence of high cholesterol levels in hypertensive patients in the Framingham Study. Am J Medicine 80(2 supp 1):23-32.
8. World Health Organization (WHO) (1982) Prevention of coronary heart disease, report of a WHO expert committee, Technical Report Series No. 678, WHO, Geneva, 53 pp.
9. Anonymous (1989) Importance of knowing HDL level emphasized. Internal Medicine News: the Leading Independent Newspaper for the Internist, November 1-14.
10. Kannel WB, Castelli WP, Gordon T (1979) Cholesterol in the prediction of atherosclerotic disease: new perspectives based on the Framingham Study. Ann Intern Med 90(1):85-91.
11. Kannel WB, Neaton JD, Wentworth D, Thomas HE, Stamler J, Hulley SB, Kjelsberg MO (1986) Overall and coronary heart disease mortality rates in relation to major risk factors in 325,348 men screened for the MRFIT (Multiple Risk Factor Intervention Trial). Amer Heart J 112(4):825-836.
12. Stamler J, Wentworth D, Neaton JD (1986) Is the relationship between serum cholesterol and risk of premature death from coronary heart disease continuous and graded? Findings in 356,222 primary screenees of the Multiple Risk Factor Intervention Trial (MRFIT). JAMA 256(2):2823-2828.

Chapter 9

1. Hayward RA, Hofer TP, Vijan S (2006) Narrative review: lack of evidence for recommended low-density lipoprotein treatment targets: a solvable problem. Ann Intern Med 145(7):520-530.
2. Fuhrmans V (2001) European panel to conduct review of cholesterol drugs. Wall Street Journal, New York, 10 August.
3. Grundy SM, Cleeman JI, Merz CN, Brewer HB Jr., Clark LT, Hunninghake DB, Pasternak RC, Smith SC Jr., Stone NJ; National Heart, Lung, and Blood Institute; American College of Cardiology Foundation; American Heart Association (2004) Implications of recent clinical trials for the National Cholesterol Education Program Adult Treatment Panel III guidelines. Circulation 110(2):227-239.
4. Baigent C, Keech A, Kearney PM, Blackwell L, Buck G, Pollicino C, Kirby A, Sourjina T, Peto R, Collins R, Simes R; Cholesterol Treatment Trialists' (CTT) Collaborators (2005) Efficacy and safety of cholesterol-lowering treatment: prospective meta-analysis of data from 90,056 participants in 14 randomized trials of statins. Lancet 366(9493):1267-1278.
5. Center for Science in the Public Interest (2004) Washington, (released 23 Sept. 2004, accessed Oct. 2006), <http://www.cspinet.org/new/200409231.html>.

6. Therapeutics Initiative (2003) Do statins have a role in primary prevention? University of British Columbia, Vancouver, (released 16 Oct. 2003, accessed Oct. 2006), <http://www.ti.ubc.ca/pages/letter48.htm>.

7. Golomb BA, Criqui MH (2006) Statin Adverse Effects. University of California San Diego Statin Effects Study Group, (updated 2 Aug. 2006, accessed Oct. 2006), <http://medicine.ucsd.edu/SES/statin_information.htm>.

8. Talbert RL (2006) Safety issues with statin therapy. J Am Pharm Assoc 46(4):479-488.

9. Davidson M, Jacobson T (2001) How statins work: the development of cardiovascular disease and its treatment with 3-hydroxy-3-methylglutaryl coenzyme A reductase inhibitors. Medscape Continuing Medical Education (CME) Professional Credit Activity.

10. Vaughan CJ, Murphy MB, Buckley BM (1996) Statins do more than just lower cholesterol. Lancet 348(9034):1079-1082.

11. Massy ZA, Keane WF, Kasiske BL (1996) Inhibition of the mevalonate pathway: benefits beyond cholesterol reduction? Lancet 347(8994):102-103.

12. Liao JK, Laufs U (2005) Pleiotropic effects of statins. Annu Rev Pharmacol Toxicol 45:89-118.

13. Kolovou G (2001) The Treatment of coronary heart disease: an update: Part 3: statins beyond cholesterol lowering. Curr Med Res Opinion 17(1):34-37.

14. Van de Wiel A, Caillard, CA (2002) Statins and the stroke-cholesterol paradox. Neth J Med 60(1):4-9.

15. Wanner C, Krane V, Marz W, Olschewski M, Mann JF, Ruf G, Ritz E (2005) Atorvastatin in patients with type 2 diabetes mellitus undergoing hemodialysis. N Eng J Med 353(3):238-248.

16. Regier, L (2006) Personal communication, Saskatoon City Hospital, 701 Queen St., Saskatoon, Sk Canada S7K0M7. See also NNTs for statins in various risk groups – major trial data (standardized for 5 years), Table 1 (available online at <http://www.rxfiles.ca/acrobat/Lipid-Q&A-Update-Oct04.pdf>).

17. American Heart Association (2006) Heart disease and stroke statistics – 2006 update. Circulation 113(6):e85-151.

Chapter 10

1. Jorgensen OD, Kronborg O, Fenger C (2002) A randomized study of screening for colorectal cancer using faecal occult blood testing: results after 13 years and seven biennial screening rounds. Gut 50(1):29-32.

2. American Cancer Society (2002) Cancer Facts & Figures 2002. ACS, Atlanta, GA, 44 pp. (available at http://www.cancer.org/docroot/STT/stt_0_2002.asp).

3. American Cancer Society (2004) Cancer Facts & Figures 2004. ACS, Atlanta, GA, 58 pp. (available at http://www.cancer.org/docroot/STT/stt_0_2004.asp).

4. U.S. Preventive Services Task Force (1996) Guide to clinical preventive services, 2nd ed. Lippincott Williams & Wilkins, Baltimore, 953 pp.

5. Mandel JS, Bond JH, Church TR, Snover DC, Bradley GM, Schuman LM, Ederer F (1993) The Minnesota colon cancer control study: reducing mortality from colorectal cancer by screening for fecal occult blood. N Engl J Med 328(19):1365-1371.
6. Hardcastle JD, Chamberlain JO, Robinson MH, Moss SM, Amar SS, Balfour TW, James PD, Mangham, CM (1996) Randomized controlled trial of faecal-occult-blood screening for colorectal cancer. Lancet 348(9040):1472-1477.
7. Kronborg O, Fenger C, Olsen J, Jorgensen OD, Sondergaard O (1996) Randomized study of screening for colorectal cancer with faecal-occult-blood test. Lancet 348(9040):1467-1471.

Chapter 11

1. National Center for Health Statistics (2005) Health, United States, 2005, with chartbook on trends in the health of Americans. U.S. Government Printing Office, Hyattsville, Maryland, 535 pp.
2. Perez-Pena, R (2003) Smoking ban relies on voluntary compliance. The New York Times, March 28.
3. Centers for Disease Control and Prevention (2002) Cigarette smoking among adults – United States, 2002. MMWR 53(20):427-431.
4. U.S. Department of Health and Human Services (2004) The health consequences of smoking: a report of the Surgeon General. U.S. Department of Health and Human Services, Centers for Disease Control and Prevention, National Center for Chronic Disease Prevention and Health Promotion, Office on Smoking and Health, Atlanta, GA, chapters available online at <www.cdc. gov>.
5. Jacobs DR, Adachi H, Mulder I, Kromhout D, Menotti A, Nissinen A, Blackburn H (1999) Cigarette smoking and mortality risk: twenty-five-year follow-up of the Seven Countries Study. Arch Intern Med 159:733-740.
6. Doll R, Peto R, Boreham J, Sutherland I (2006) Mortality in relation to smoking: 50 years' observations on male British doctors. BMJ 328(7455):1519-1527.

Chapter 12

1. U.S. Environmental Protection Agency (2003) Water on tap: what you need to know, EPA 816-K-03-007. Office of Water, Washington, D.C., 32 pp. (also available online at http://www.epa.gov/safewater/wot/index.html).
2. Madigan MT, Martinko JM (2006) Brock biology of microorganisms, 11th ed. Pearson Prentice Hall, Upper Saddle River, NJ, 1088 pp.
3. Maier RM, Pepper IL, Gerba CP (2000) Environmental microbiology. Academic Press, San Diego, CA, 585 pp.

4. Brody H, Rip MR, Vinten-Johansen P, Paneth N, Rachman S (2000) Map-making and myth-making in Broad Street: the London cholera epidemic, 1854. Lancet 356:64-68.

5. McGhee TJ (1991) Water supply and sewerage, 6th ed. McGraw-Hill, Inc., New York, NY, 704 pp.

6. Centers for Disease Control (2004) Surveillance for waterborne disease outbreaks associated with drinking water - United States 2001-2002. MMWR Surveillance Summaries 53(SS08):23-45.

7. Viessman W Jr., Hammer MJ (2005) Water supply and pollution control, 7th ed. Pearson Prentice Hall, Upper Saddle River, NJ, 876 pp.

8. World Health Organization and United Nations Children's Fund (2000) Global Water supply and sanitation assessment 2000 report. WHO/UNICEF, Geneva, 80 pp. (document also available online at http://www.who.int/water_sanitation_health/monitoring/globalassess/en/).

9. Montgomery MA, Elimelech M (2007) Water and sanitation in developing countries: including health in the equation. Env Sci Tech 41(1):17-24.

10. U.S. Environmental Protection Agency (2002) List of drinking water contaminants and MCLs. (accessed September 2006 at http://www.epa.gov/safewater/contaminants/index.html).

11. National Research Council (2004) Review of the Army's technical guides on assessing and managing chemical hazards to deployed personnel. National Academy Press, Washington, D.C., 195 pp.

Chapter 13

1. National Research Council (NRC) (1999) Health effects of exposure to radon. Committee on the Health Risks of Exposure to Radon (BEIR VI), National Academy Press, Washington, D.C., 487 pp.

2. Samet JM (1997) Epidemiologic studies of ionizing radiation and cancer: past successes and future challenges. Environmental Health Perspectives 105(4):883-889.

3. Donohue K, Royal H (1996) Importance of radon as a threat to public health. Otolaryngol Head Neck Surg 114:271-276.

4. Mendez D, Warner KE, Courant PN (1998) Effects of radon mitigation vs. smoking cessation in reducing radon-related risk of lung cancer. Am J Public Health 88(5):811-812.

5. Pawel DJ, Puskin JS (2004) The U.S. Environmental Protection Agency's assessment of risks from indoor radon. Health Physics 87(1):68-74.

6. Tracy BL, Krewski D, Chen J, Zielinski JM, Brand KP, Meyerhof D (2006) Assessment and management of residential radon health risks: a report from the Health Canada radon workshop. J of Toxicology and Environmental Health, Part A 69:735-738.

7. Environmental Protection Agency (EPA) (2005) A Citizen's guide to radon: a guide to protecting yourself and your family from radon, www.epa.gov/radon/pubs/citguide.html.
8. Krewski D, Rai SN, Zielinski JM, Hopke PK (1999) Characterization of uncertainty and variability in residential radon cancer risks. Annals New York Academy of Sciences 895:245-272.

Chapter 14

1. Lackey RL (1997) Ecological risk analysis. In: Molak V (ed.) Fundamentals of risk analysis and risk management. CRC Press, Boca Raton, pp. 87-97.
2. U.S. Environmental Protection Agency (1992) Framework for ecological risk assessment: EPA/630/R-92/001. US EPA Risk Assessment Forum, Washington, D.C., 41 pp.
3. Environmental Defense Fund (1997) News Release: 25 years after DDT ban, Bald Eagles, Osprey numbers soar. (available online at http://www.environmentaldefense. org/pressrelease.cfm?contentID=2446).
4. Center for Environmental and Regulatory Information Systems (1993) Spotted knapweed: fact sheet. US Department of Agriculture Animal and Plant Health Inspection Service (APHIS), Plant Protection and Quarantine (PPQ), Cooperative Agricultural Pest Survey (CAPS), (available online at http://www.ceris. purdue.edu/napis/index.html).
5. Evans EW (1993) Biological control agents for Utah weeds: the Knapweed seedhead gall flies – Entomology fact sheet no. 91. Utah State University Extension Service, Logan, UT, 4 pp.
6. Pearson DE, Callaway RM (2006) Biological control agents elevate hantavirus by subsidizing deer mouse populations. Ecol Lett 9(4):443-450.
7. Moran PJ (1988) Crown-of-thorns Starfish questions and answers. Australian Institute of Marine Science (AIMS), Queensland, 198 pp. (also available at http://www.aims.gov.au/pages/reflib/cot-starfish/pages/cot-000.html).

Chapter 15

1. National Research Council (2004) Nonnative oysters in the Chesapeake Bay. The National Academies Press, Washington D.C., 326 pp.
2. Kennedy VS, Breisch LL (1983) Sixteen decades of political management of the oyster fishery in Maryland's Chesapeake Bay. J Envir Man 16(2): 153-171.
3. NOAA Chesapeake Bay Office (2004) Native oysters. (available online at <http://noaa.chesapeakebay.net/NativeOysters.aspx>).

4. Rothschild BJ, Ault JS, Goulletquer P, Heral, M (1994) Decline of the Chesapeake Bay oyster population: a century of habitat destruction and overfishing. Mar Ecol Prog Ser 111(1-2):29-39.

5. Burreson EM, Stokes NA, Friedman CS (2000) Increased virulence in an introduced pathogen: *Haplosporidium nelsoni* (MSX) in the Eastern oyster *Crassostrea virginica*. J Aquat Anim Health 12(1):1-8.

6. Ford SE, Tripp MR (1996) Diseases and defense mechanisms. In: Kennedy VS, Newell RIE, Eble AF (eds) The Eastern oyster: *Crassostrea virginica*. Maryland Sea Grant College Program Publication UM-SG-TS-96-01, College Park, pp. 581-660.

7. Kennedy VS, Newell RIE, Eble AF (eds) (1996) The Eastern oyster: *Crassostrea virginica*. Maryland College Sea Grant Program Publication UM-SG-TS-96-01, College Park, 772 pp.

8. Haskin HH, Andrews JD (1988) Uncertainties and speculations about the life cycle of the Eastern oyster pathogen *Haplosporidium nelsoni* (MSX). In: Fisher WS (ed) Disease processes in marine bivalve mollusks. American Fisheries Society Special Publication 18, Bethesda, Maryland, pp. 5-22.

9. Carlton JT (2001) Introduced species in U.S. coastal waters: environmental impacts and management priorities. Pew Oceans Commission, Arlington, Virginia, 36 pp.

10. Sindermann CJ (1990) Principal diseases of marine fish and shellfish, 2nd ed., Academic Press, San Diego, 516 pp.

11. Hayak FA (1991) Economic freedom. Basil Blackwell, Oxford, p. 287.

12. Latin H (1997) Science, regulation, and toxic risk assessment. In: Molak, V (ed) Fundamentals of risk analysis and risk management. Lewis Publishers, Boca Raton, 472 pp.

Chapter 16

1. Maryland Department of the Environment (2004) Water quality analyses of chromium in the Inner Harbor/Northwest Branch and Bear Creek portions of Baltimore Harbor in Baltimore City and Baltimore County, Maryland: Report to EPA Region III, MDE, Baltimore, 16 pp.

2. McGee BK, Fisher DJ, Yonkos LT, Ziegler GP, Turley S (1999) Assessment of sediment contamination, acute toxicity, and population viability of the estuarine amphipod *Leptocheirus plumulosus* in Baltimore Harbor, Maryland. Environ Toxicol Chem 18(10):2151-2160.

3. U.S. Environmental Protection Agency (2004) The incidence and severity of sediment contamination in the surface waters of the United States, National Sediment Quality Survey, 2nd ed., EPA-823-R-04-007. Office of Science and Technology, Washington, D.C., 280 pp.

4. National Research Council (2003) Bioavailability of contaminants in soils and sediments: processes, tools, and applications. National Academies Press, Washington, D.C., 432 pp.

5. Evanko CR, Dzombak DA (1997) Remediation of metals-contaminated soils and groundwater, technology evaluation report TE-97-01. Ground-Water Remediation Technologies Analysis Center (GWRTAC), Pittsburgh, PA, 53 pp.
6. Rifkin E, Gwinn P, Bouwer EJ (2004) Chromium and sediment toxicity. Environ Toxicol Chem 38(14):276A-271A.
7. Boothman WS, Berry WJ, Serbst JR, Edwards PA (2000) Predicting toxicity of chromium-spiked sediments by using acid-volatile sulfide and interstitial water measurements. US EPA, National Health and Environmental Effects Research Laboratory, Atlantic Ecology Division, Narragansett, RI. Presented at: 6th Annual NAC/SETAC Conference, Newport, Rhode Island, April 2000.
8. Berry WJ, Boothman WS, Serbst JR, Edwards PA (2002) Effects of chromium in sediment: 1. toxicity tests with saltwater field sediments. US EPA, National Health and Environmental Effects Research Laboratory, Atlantic Ecology Division, Narragansett, RI. Presented at: SETAC 23rrd Annual Meeting, Salt Lake City, Utah, 16-20 November 2002.
9. Wang W, Griscom SB, Fisher NS (1997) Bioavailability of Cr(III) and Cr(VI) to marine mussels from solute and particulate pathways. Environ Sci Technol 31(2):603-611.
10. Agency for Toxic Substances and Disease Registry (2000) Toxicological profile for chromium. US Department of Health and Human Services, ATSDR, Atlanta, Georgia, (available online at < http://www.atsdr.cdc.gov/>).
11. US Environmental Protection Agency (1985) Ambient water quality criteria for chromium-1984, EPA 440/5-84-029. Office of Water, Washington, D.C., 99 pp.
12. Brumbaugh WG, May TW, Wiedmeyer RH, Besser JM, Ingersoll CG (2002) Effects of chromium in sediment: 4. monitoring of chromium in sediment, pore water, and overlying water of Cr(VI) spiked freshwater sediments. U.S Geological Survey. Presented at: SETAC 23rd Annual Meeting Salt Lake City, Utah, 16-20 November 2002.

Chapter 17

1. Gotzsche PC, Olsen O (2000) Is screening for breast cancer with mammography justifiable? Lancet 355(9198):129-134.
2. Tabar L, Yen MF, Vitak B, Chen HH, Smith RA, Duffy SW (2003) Mammog-raphy service screening and mortality in breast cancer patients: 20-year follow-up before and after introduction of screening. Lancet 361(9367):1405-1410.
3. The lifetime risk data mentioned throughout this chapter is available online from the National Cancer Institute (www.nci.gov) and the National Institutes of Health (www.nih.gov).

Chapter 18

1. Environmental Protection Agency (2005) A citizen's guide to radon: a guide to protecting yourself and your family from radon, EPA 402-K-02-006. EPA, Indoor Environments Division, Washington, D.C., 16 pp, (also available online at <www.epa.gov/radon/pubs/citguide.html>).

2. US Food and Drug Administration (1973) Compounds used in food-producing animals, procedures for determining acceptability of assay methods used for assuring the absence of residues in edible products of such animals. Proposed rule, Federal Register, July 19:19226-19230.

3. Kelly KE (1991) The myth of 10^{-6} as a definition of acceptable risk. (Updated from a paper originally presented at the 84th annual meeting of the Air & Waste Management Association, Vancouver, B.C., Canada, June 16-21, 1991).

4. Howe HL, Wu X, Ries LA, Cokkinides V, Ahmed F, Jemal A, Miller B, Williams M, Ward E, Wingo PA, Ramirez A, Edwards BK (2006) Annual report to the nation on the status of cancer, 1975-2003, featuring cancer among U.S. Hispanic/Latino populations. Cancer 107(8):1711-1742.

5. Kiberstis PA, Travis J (2006) Celebrating a glass half-full. Science 312(5777):1157.

6. National Cancer Institute (2001) PLCO cancer screening trial completes recruitment. (Dated 26 July 2001, accessed Oct. 2006 at http://www.cancer.gov/newscenter/plcopr/).

7. American Cancer Society (accessed 10/18/2006) Overview: prostate cancer. (available at <http://www.cancer.org/docroot/CRI/CRI 2_1x.asp?dt=36>).

8. Jacobsen SL, Katusic SK, Bergstralh EJ, Oesterling JE, Ohrt D, Klee GG, Chute CG, Lieber MM (1995) Incidence of prostate cancer diagnosis in the eras before and after serum prostate-specific antigen testing. JAMA 274(18):1445-1449.

9. Crawford ED, DeAntoni EP, Etzioni R, Schaefer VC, Olsen RM, Ross CA (1996) Serum prostate-specific antigen and digital rectal examination for early detection of prostate cancer in a national community-based program, The Prostate Cancer Education Council. Urology 47(6):863-869.

10. Zoorob R, Anderson R, Cefalu C, Sidani M (2001) Cancer screening guidelines. Am Fam Physician 63(6):1101-1112.

11. Harris R, Lohr KN (2002) Screening for prostate cancer: an update of the evidence for the United States Preventative Services Task Force. Ann Intern Med 137(11):917-929.

12. Andriole GL, Levin DL, Crawford ED, Gelmann EP, Pinsky PF, Chia D, Kramer BS, Reding D, Church TR, Grubb RL, Izmirlian G, Ragard LR, Clapp JD, Prorok PC, Gohagan JK; PLCO Project Team (2005) Prostate cancer screening in the prostate, lung, colorectal and ovarian (PLCO) cancer screening trial: findings from the initial screening round of a randomized trial. JCNI 97(6):433-438.

Appendix A

1. Bowker AH, Lieberman GJ (1972) Engineering statistics, 2nd ed. Prentice-Hall, Englewood Cliffs, NJ, 641 pp.
2. Olive JD, Clark VA (1974) Applied statistics: analysis of variance and regression. John Wiley & Sons, New York, NY, 387 pp.
3. Williams PRD, Paustenbach, DJ (2002) Chapter 5: Risk characterization. In: Paustenbach DJ (ed) Human and ecological risk assessment: theory and practice, pp. 293-366.
4. Morgan MG, Henrion M (1990) Uncertainty: a guide to dealing with uncertainty in quantitative risk and policy analysis. Cambridge University Press, Cambridge, England, 332 pp.
5. Cullen AC, Small MJ (2004) Uncertain risk: the role and limits of quantitative assessment. In: McDaniels T, Small MJ (eds) Risk analysis and society: an interdisciplinary characterization of the field. Cambridge University Press, Cambridge, United Kingdom, pp. 163-212.
6. Ramaswami A, Milford JB, Small, MJ (2005) Integrated environmental modeling: pollutant transport, fate, and risk in the environment. John Wiley and Sons, Inc., Hoboken, NJ, 678 pp.

Appendix B

1. Kannel WB, Castelli WP, Gordon T (1979) Cholesterol in the prediction of atherosclerotic disease: new perspectives based on the Framingham Study. Ann Intern Med 90(1):85-91.
2. Kannel WB, Neaton JD, Wentworth D, Thomas HE, Stamler J, Hulley SB, Kjelsberg MO (1986) Overall and coronary heart disease mortality rates in relation to major risk factors in 325,348 men screened for the MRFIT (Multiple Risk Factor Intervention Trial). Amer Heart J 112(4):825-836.
3. Stamler J, Wentworth D, Neaton JD (1986) Is the relationship between serum cholesterol and risk of premature death from coronary heart disease continuous and graded? Findings in 356,222 primary screenees of the Multiple Risk Factor Intervention Trial (MRFIT). JAMA 256(2):2823-2828.
4. Centers for Disease Control and Prevention (2003) Cholesterol status among adults in the United States, national health and nutrition examination survey. National Center for Health Statistics, Hyattsville, MD, (available online at <http://www.cdc.gov/nchs/data/nhanes/databriefs/adultcholesterol.pdf>).

Index

About the Authors

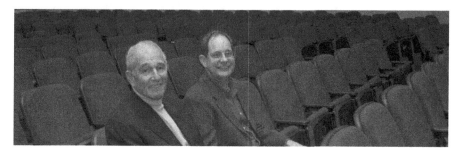

Authors Erik Rifkin and Edward Bouwer

Erik Rifkin is the president of an environmental consulting firm in Baltimore, MD that specializes in the characterization of ecological and human health risks from exposure to contaminants in soil, water, air, and sediments. His firm provides assistance and guidance to federal and state regulatory agencies and corporations regarding the nature and magnitude of environmental risks and potential remediation strategies. Dr. Rifkin's broad experience includes the communication of health risks and benefits to groups concerned with these issues.

Edward J. Bouwer is Professor of Environmental Engineering at Johns Hopkins University in Baltimore, Maryland. He has extensive experience with water and soil pollution and treatment. His research provides guidance on defining and managing environmental risks and how to interpret human and ecological health risk data. Dr. Bouwer has served on several National Research Council committees that provide guidance on managing human and ecological risks to Congress, regulatory agencies, and the scientific community.

Guest author **Bob Sheff**, MD, received his medical training as a radiologist at UCLA and Johns Hopkins Medical Center. He spent his career practicing medicine and running one of the largest medical managed-care systems in the United States. Now semi-retired, he devotes his time to helping non-profit organizations and individual people address their medical concerns. He lives in Columbia, Maryland.